Rituals of Birth

RITUALS of BIRTH

From Prehistory to the Present

Ann Warren Turner

DAVID McKAY COMPANY, INC.
NEW YORK

COPYRIGHT © 1978 by Ann Warren Turner

All rights reserved, including the right to reproduce this book, or parts thereof, in any form, except for the inclusion of brief quotations in a review.

Library of Congress Cataloging in Publication Data

Turner, Ann Warren.
Rituals of birth.

Includes index.
SUMMARY: Describes childbirth customs in different cultures throughtout history.
1. Birth (in religion, folk-lore, etc.)
2. Childbirth. [1. Birth (in religion, folk-lore, etc.) 2. Childbirth]
I. Title.
GN482.1.T87   392'.12   77-14904
ISBN 0-679-20440-7

10 9 8 7 6 5 4 3 2 1
MANUFACTURED IN THE UNITED STATES OF AMERICA

CONTENTS

BIRTH IN PREHISTORY	1
Ice Age Mystery	3
BIRTH IN ANCIENT TIMES	9
A Mother of Sons	11
BIRTH IN HUNTING/GATHERING CULTURES	21
Two Mothers	23
That My Hood Be Full	33
BIRTH IN AN AGRICULTURAL TRIBE	41
The Middle Place	43
BIRTH IN URBAN CULTURES	53
My Thousand Ounces of Gold	55
Birth of the Sun-King	63
MULTIPLE BIRTHS	73
Strange Birth	75
The Fearful Ones	81
BIRTH IN MODERN TIMES	91
Birth in America	93
THE POPULATION PROBLEM: BOTH SIDES	105
Contraception Through History	107
How to Get a Child	119
GLOSSARY	127
FOR FURTHER READING	135
INDEX	139

"Every human society is faced not with one population problem but with two; how to beget and rear enough children and how not to beget and rear too many." [1]

---

[1] Margaret Mead, *Male and Female* (New York: Dell Publishing Co., Inc., 1968), pp. 224–25.

Birth in Prehistory

Chapter 1
ICE AGE MYSTERY

> *Time:* The last
> Ice Age, 30,000–
> 10,000 B.C.
> *Place:* Russia, to Central
> and Western Europe.
> *Characters:* Cro-Magnon men
> and women

This is a detective story. For much of archaeology is detective work, piecing together a clue here, a clue there to get a picture of how people lived in tribes and times long ago.

We are going to go far back in our hunt for clues, back to the last Ice Age. What we are searching for are bones, carvings, paintings on cave walls, remains of huts and homes, and ashes from ancient fires. What can they tell us? These scattered finds will show how people lived in that harsh age and, hopefully, will let us know something about women and how they gave birth.

The first find is a 21,000-year-old limestone block from a cave in France. On the block is a carving of a fat woman with hanging breasts, a large belly, and swelling thighs. She is like other female images of the Ice Age and may be an ancient goddess who was linked to the moon. In her right hand she holds a horn, and on the horn are thirteen marks. The archaeologist Alexander Marshack thinks these symbolize one lunar year, thirteen rounds of the moon's waxing and waning. What does this tell us? This and other man-made objects of the Ice Age led Marshack to believe that ancient men and women could measure time and that they marked down the moon's cycles and the different seasons in their carvings and sculpture. How does this relate to women and pregnancy? If Ice Age people could note time, then they probably linked women's menstrual cycles to the moon. The cycles tend to last twenty-eight to thirty days, about the span from the first to next new crescent of the moon. The length of a pregnancy could also be predicted if people told time by the moon; ten lunar months equals a pregnancy. We can imagine a woman, dressed in skins, making a mark for the first period she missed. Nine more notches would take her to the time of her delivery and she could then say to her husband: "The child will come in the moon-of-returning-reindeer"; or, "The child will be born during the moon-of-disappearing-salmon."

This is the first clue in the mystery: men and women of the last Ice Age could measure time; they possibly linked a woman's menstrual cycle to the moon, and may have predicted the length of a pregnancy.

The next piece of evidence is a series of carvings of womens' breasts. Sometimes these tiny objects (usually of ivory or bone) have holes in the back. A sinew or strip of hide could be put through it and the image hung around the neck. Other carvings are without holes and possibly were held in the hands. Both may have been used as protection against barrenness, or as magic charms to help with childbearing and nursing. They may represent an ancient goddess, the same one shown in the figurines of fat women. As some Christian women today might look at a statue of the Madonna and pray for a child, an Ice Age woman might have touched a breast carving and murmured; "Mother, fill my body with a child"; or, "Mother, protect me in my time of bearing."

The third find is hard to interpret. Throughout the last Ice Age people carved the signs for a woman's vulva on cave walls, on bones, on abstracted female forms, and on small circles of bone and stone. We don't know if these carvings were held, worn around the neck, or used in some ritual way. They might symbolize one part of myths told about the ancient, life-giving goddess (as Marshack suggests), maybe relating to the menstrual cycle. Or they and other vulva signs could represent "the doorway of a new life," [1] the place of birth. Imagine a small band of Ice Age hunters and their wives and children sitting around the fire at night, listening to tales of an all-powerful goddess. A pregnant woman among them might be comforted and reassured by those stories. "She gave birth to mankind, so I, too, will bear my children safely and easily."

The fourth clue is a group of fascinating carvings. They are of stylized women, reduced to curving bodies with enormous buttocks and bent knees. Some images were hung around the neck; others are palm-sized and seem made to be held. Were these strange images used by women during labor? Did some Ice Age women squat or kneel, clutching a curved figurine, and say, "Mother, help me now, be with me during this birth"? We don't know; this is a mystery with no foreseeable answer.

The last piece of evidence is this: small sculptures of fat women are sometimes found buried near the remains of Ice Age hearths. A typical figurine has abundant breasts, belly, and large thighs. To this author, she looks like a mother, a bearer of many. Is she a figure of an Ice Age goddess? Since these carved women are often buried near hearths, could they be guardians of the fire so vital in those cold, harsh times? If you had a magnifying glass in one hand, you might discover bits of red coloring on some of the images. They are the remains of red ocher (a natural earth pigment) often smeared on the dead during the last Ice Age. The coloring is a symbol of life and vitality, of power. We can imagine a hunter of 20,000 years ago, rubbing the red earth on the carvings. Perhaps it represented birth-blood to him and to others and increased the goddess's power as the life-giving mother of human and animal young.

[1] Margaret Mead, *Male and Female* (New York: Dell Publishing Co., 1968), p. 230.

As detectives with a series of clues, what can we say about the evidence? We think a female goddess was worshipped and tales were told about her. Possibly those stories spoke of how she was linked to the moon; how her vulva was the seat of new life; how her breasts gave suck; and how her curved, fleshy body gave birth to mankind and all life.

But what about the real women of the last Ice Age? What can we say about their experience with pregnancy and birth?

They probably had some idea of how children were conceived. We know they did not say, as we do; "The man's sperm travels up the woman's Fallopian tubes and there pierces the ripe ovum"; for that is knowledge only gained in the last century with the help of microscopes. But they may have said; "The husband enters his wife and puts the soul of the child inside"; or, "The father gives the bones to the child, while the mother grows the flesh." These are the kinds of explanations sometimes made by modern hunting tribes.

When time came for the child to be born, did women stay in the hut or go outside to a temporary brush shelter? We don't know; there aren't enough clues. But we can look to modern hunting tribes to see what they do. Often, women's blood is thought to be dangerous to men, the hunters. When a woman gives birth, it must be outside, away from the men. In the last Ice Age, the sisters and female relatives of a pregnant woman might have said, "Come quickly, outside to the birth hut." Or women could have told the men, "Out, get away, her time has begun." If the hearth was sacred to women, the wife might have taken a position by the fire, ready to deliver. Yet the Polar Eskimos are a hunting people and do not separate their men from women giving birth. The husband even helps push the baby out of the mother. So Ice Age hunters may have stroked their wives' backs and helped during the time of labor.

Did women squat, kneel, or lie down during birth? Probably women in different tribes and times had varying customs. There is only one clue to the birth-position of Ice Age women and that is the "buttocks carvings" of women with bent knees; they may represent the delivery position. Perhaps a woman half-squattered for the birth, holding onto a strip of hide that hung from the hut's roof. Or women may have knelt during labor, with female helpers supporting her on either side.

As the baby slid out, was it allowed to fall to the ground? Maybe a pile of skins cushioned its fall, or other women received the child in their hands. Someone probably wiped the child dry with skins or soft grasses and either bit through or cut the navel cord with a flint tool.

Then the placenta, that magical sac of flesh and blood, followed the baby. A woman might have taken it outside and left it for the wild animals. Or perhaps someone scooped a hole in the earth by the fire and buried the afterbirth. If the hearth was sacred to women and to a guardian goddess, maybe a charm or prayer was chanted over the placenta as it was buried: "Mother, guard this boy and make him a great hunter"; or, "Mother, protect this girl and make her a bearer of many." So the North American Nootka Indians sang their wishes for the new child over the afterbirth.

This stranger, the newborn, would then need to be welcomed into the family, made "one of us." For even in the simplest of cultures, people distinguish between "them" (the people outside the tribe) and "us" (family and relatives). The father or a female relative might have held the child up to the fire, "introducing" him or her to the guardian of the house and tribe. Perhaps they smeared red ocher on the new one to make the child a relative, or to put it under the protection of the fat goddess who herself was covered with red.

How was the child named? In some American Indian tribes of the last century, a child was not named until he was older (6–8 years) and had shown some special trait or skill. Perhaps Ice Age hunters waited and then named their children after individual qualities; "He-of-the-stumbling-walk"; "She-of-the-fleet-foot"; "Salmon-fishing-boy"; or

"Egg-hunting girl." In other hunting tribes, names may be given to the young by the very old, or a name can be inherited from a dead relative. Then the qualities of the ancestor are believed to be passed on to the new child with the name.

Our mystery is still unsolved; only bits and pieces are known. Maybe you will be one of the detectives to kneel in the dirt, searching for bone shards and the edge of a carving. Or with your eye over the microscope, you'll examine earth from an ancient house site and say, "Those are traces from a fire where animal bones were burned." Or, "Those are remains of many wild grass seeds; these people collected and ate such seeds." We need more detectives, and we need more evidence to tell us of the lives of our ancestors so long ago—to tell us about the women who prayed and sang to a goddess, who squatted or knelt during birth, and who called their children by names we will never know.

Birth in Ancient Times

Chapter 2
A MOTHER OF SONS

Time: 432 B.C.
Place: Athens, Greece
Characters: A well-to-do Greek family

I had gone to the temple to pray and sacrifice, as I did so often those days, and was returning home with my slave woman. All along the narrow, noisy streets I looked for a bird to fly by on my right, and listened closely to the speech of passers-by. My eyes and ears were always open for omens then: the flight of a bird; the cast of the wind; a night's sigh; anything that would foretell a child would be born to me.

I had been five years without issue—five long, barren years with no son or daughter to show for it. By Demeter, no one can know what a sorrow that is, to be homeless in your husband's house. The slave girls had more importance than I, barren as I was like some bitter salt lake where no fish or eel lives. For what is a wife without children? Indeed, what is a husband without children? I knew, as Isaeus, my husband did, that a father's spirit must have a son to tend it. Only a male child can make the tomb offerings, the good things that please the dead. And only sons and daughters can keep a family alive. That is why custom says a man must marry and have children; otherwise, his name and house would cease to be. A family without children is like an olive tree without leaves—it will surely die before summer's end.

So it was not just for myself that I desired sons and

daughters, but also for Isaeus, that his name might live on. I also hoped that when we were old we would have children to care for us. As our laws say, sons and daughters must care for their aged parents, just as we cared for my husband's mother—a widow named Philotis. No one wants to reach the age of watery eyes and shaking knees without a younger one to lean on.

Philotis often asked me if I'd offended a goddess in some way. "Did you make the proper sacrifices, Demetria?" I do not think she meant to hurt me, but those questions and sharp looks only made me more silent, more alone in my husband's house.

For I had done all I could. I prayed and sacrificed to Eileithyia, she who brings children, more times than I can count. Honey cakes, wine, oil and incense I laid on her altars. She was not the only goddess to receive my gifts. I sacrificed often to Artemis, the All-Mother, asking for a child. I even remembered to pray for delivery of the babe, that I would not be like the poor woman who carried her child full three years, all because she forgot to ask the gods for deliverance of her child.

I was a willing member of the Thesmophoria, the great autumn festival for Demeter, goddess of fields and harvest. I cannot tell all I know, for they are sacred rites, but I have been down in the dark caves where the serpent lives. I have brought back the sacrificed pigs and mixed them with seed grain to scatter on the fields. I thought that if only I could touch Demeter's magic, then I, too, might be fertile—as her fields and crops are. Is not a woman like a rich field and her husband the sower? By the All-Mother, I was sowed but no life grew in me.

In my sorrow, I once thought of getting nurse to bring me an abandoned child. I'd heard how it was done. The babies are left in baskets or clay pots in some wild place, or in a god's temple. There they will die, unless some kind person takes them home. Those are the children a father cannot afford to rear, or for some reason, will not allow into the family. I've heard of women who take such babes as their own. The wife pretends to be big with child (pillows will do that), and that her time of delivery is near. The husband is put away from the women's quarters, while the nurse smuggles the baby upstairs in a pot, the child's mouth stuffed with rags to silence it. Then the babe is brought out, washed, and slapped to make it cry. Nurse runs to tell the father it's a boy or a girl, and the child is held up as if it's newborn.

I did think of it but knew I could never do such a thing. I always was a poor liar and hated pretending. Besides, a husband must be dull-witted indeed to be fooled by such a trick! And I still hoped for a child; I was not yet certain I was barren.

I do not know what turned the goddess's ear to me, or why a child at last began to grow inside. For it did happen, six years after my marriage—six long summers after the day I came to my husband's house, wearing my marriage crown and carrying the red pomegranate [a symbol of fertility] in my hand.

I may speak calmly of it now, but then I was so taken with joy, I was as a winged god. If I were not held onto, I might fly off into the sun-drenched sky.

"Now I will be justified," I said to my old nurse, "now my husband will trust me and give me place in his affairs."

"That is so, mistress," she answered. "When a wife bears a child, then the husband turns more often to her, giving her honor."

And without a child? The only honor a wife can hope for is to be left in peace, away from the disappointed eyes of her family.

During the time I carried the child, I was not picky, as some women are. I did not ask for this or that and say, "Husband! I must have eels from the river," or, "Husband! Get me some new figs!" Oh, once, I did ask for Persian apples; I had a craving for them. But that was all. I was more interested in seeing which way the babe leaned inside me. Some days it leaned to the left, meaning it would be a girl. Other days the babe was on the right side, and I thought I would have a son.

At the time of the spring harvest, the child decided to

come into the world. Philotis hurried me upstairs to the women's quarters. She laid me down on the bed, put a light coverlet over me, and sent the slave girl for the midwives. They must have been ready, for they came to the house before my second pain. The midwives were older women of good reputation, neighbors and friends who had assisted at many births before. One of the women came with a bag full of herbs.

"These are powerful herbs, daughter," she said to me as she placed them around my bed. "They are called the hand of the mother of god and will speed your delivery."

While the midwife tended me, Philotis bustled around the room crying, "Any knots here? Are all in the room free of knots?" For a tied cloth, crossed fingers or legs, even a closed hand can keep the babe from being born.

Then she came to me and unclenched my fists, saying, "Demetria, you know better than that! Will you keep the child in the womb? Remember Heracles' birth!"

So I kept my hands open, even when the pains came, remembering the story. Eileithyia, the divine midwife, prevented the hero's birth when she sat outside the birth room, closing her hands, crossing all fingers and repeating charms. Only through a trick was she made to stand up, thus releasing Heracles from his mother's womb.

With all things auspicious in the birth room, we called on the divine midwives: "Eileithyia, come to this good woman's aid"; and, "Artemis, be with us now!" I hoped Eileithyia was in the room with me, for the pains were fierce and close together now. The goddess's open hand, placed over the unborn child, would speed and ease the delivery. And Artemis, the All-Mother, would make the babe slide out.

"Help me up now," I asked the midwives, and they supported me over to the birth stool that waited beside the bed. I crouched on it, with two midwives holding my arms; one of them pressed her hand on my stomach to push the child out. Philotis kneeled in front of the birth stool, ready to catch the child as it appeared. A strange voice that could not be my own cried, "It's coming!" and below me I saw a head of black hair, a squalling face, and Philotis gently took hold of the baby's head. Then the shoulders slipped out, and the child was born into his grandmother's hands. Philotis held him up for me to see, all the time crowing, "It's a son, a son!" as if she'd just borne him herself.

One of the midwives cut the cord, while another helped me to my bed. A third was busy with the bath, putting water into a basin and making sure it was just warm enough. Philotis gave her my son, and they washed away the birthblood, unlucky as it was. The babe seemed to enjoy it, the funny thing, kicking his feet out and opening his eyes wide. Then the midwives patted him dry, rubbed his body with olive oil, and swaddled him from his feet to his neck with a thin band of wool. At last they gave me my son to suckle.

While he was trying to suck—and it surprised me how quick he was—nurse came up to the bedside.

"Have you forgotten?" she asked quietly.

We were so taken with the babe, we'd not made the sign against the burning eye. It was nurse who spat on her fingers and rubbed my son's forehead. That would protect him from the evil eye that makes young babes sicken and die.

It was hard for me to imagine then, tired as I was, that the Fates were also in the birthroom. I could not see them, of course; that is not granted to us. But I knew the three sisters were there: Klotho, who spins life's thread; Lachesis, who measures it out; and Atropos, who cuts the thread at life's end. I wondered how long the fate line would be for my son. Long enough to grow into a man? Long enough to fight in the endless wars of Athens? Long enough for him to marry and have children, so one day I would be cared for as I now cared for Philotis?

But my mind was too tired to think much on these things. With the long night's labor over, and with Apollo's light streaming in on my son's face, I slept.

I woke to Isaeus, my husband, who leaned over me with a smile as wide as the Greek harbor. It almost frightened me to see him so happy.

"I've put the wreath of olive leaves on the street door, Demetria, so all will know our son is born. And I smeared pitch on the doorway," he added. That would keep evil ones from entering and harming the child.

My husband had rare words of praise for me that day: "A fine wife, to be the mother of sons!" And about the boy: "Our son is more beautiful than the dawn; he has cloud-gray eyes."

When nurse heard him praising the boy, she held up her hand and said, "Ssst, sst! Quiet now, no more of that! You'll bring down bad luck on your babe if you praise him too highly. You know that." She looked reprovingly at Isaeus.

He shrugged his shoulders, embarrassed as a small boy, and tried to undo the damage by saying bad things of our child.

"Ah, he's an ill-favored lout, the wrinkled wretch! How could a father be proud of such a toad?" and he clucked disapprovingly.

Nurse added to his words with, "He's a puny mouse! Your mother must have drunk vinegar for nine months to make such a sour-faced babe!"

I hated to hear such words about my beautiful son, but it must be done. Making nothing of the child and saying he was ill-favored would keep away the envy and jealousy of the gods.

For this was a dangerous time, between the birth and the fifth-day ceremony when the child would be put under the protection of the household gods. Now the babe was unprotected, nameless, prey to the malice of witches. I shuddered to think of them, the dread women who come to suck a babe's lifeblood. Mormo might sneak into the room at night and feed on my son. She was insatiable and devoured others' children, having already lost her own. Or the strix could fasten her teeth on my child, leaving him pale and drawn the next day.

Nurse, with her calm sense, chanted the charm to keep away the blood-sucking monster. I heard the magic words, "to send away the strix, the crier by night, from the land, the nameless bird, upon the swift ships."[1]

Finally, the fifth day after the birth came—five days of anxious waiting, charms, and prayers to the gods and goddesses for protection.

Downstairs, in the main living room, our close relatives were gathered. They must be there, as the ceremony would make the babe part of our family, part of them too.

On the hearth the bright flames leapt up, sacred to Hestia. My husband's bare skin glowed in the light, as did mine and our other naked relatives. Holding the bare child to his warm skin, Isaeus ran swiftly around the fire and we followed. As he ran, the strangeness of the newborn was blown away and the babe was purified by the fire. By clasping the child to him, Isaeus said to all: "I will be father to this child, I will rear him as my son." For until the running around, a father could abandon or expose the baby.

I will never forget it—the swift running, the silent child, and the warm fire cleansing the babe and all of us who had touched the dangerous blood of birth. Now the boy was a part of the family and protected by Hestia and our household gods.

For the next few days, Isaeus and I argued about the child's name.

"I think he should be called Lysanias," I said boldly. Now I was a mother, I had more courage. "My grandfather was a great soldier of the Persian Wars."

"War-maker!" Isaeus snorted. "I want him named Theagenes, a lucky name. Did not *my* grandfather build the steps of the Parthenon? It was his trade and his money that did that!"

I lifted my head, saying no to a mere merchant's name. And so it went, back and forth, until we settled on Apollodōrus, after the god, of course. Apollo was my

---

[1] William R. Halliday, *Greek and Roman Folklore* (New York: Cooper Square Publishers, 1963), p. 33.

husband's chosen god, and I remembered how his brilliant light shone on my newborn's face. Apollodōrus he would be.

The tenth day after the birth came, a clear sunny day that matched my son's name. All our relatives, along with our good friends, were invited for the naming and the feast. Downstairs in the living room with the hearth, Isaeus stood with the child in his arms. Surrounded by kin and friends, he called out, "I name this boy Apollodōrus." There was a murmur of agreement and approval from the company. "A fine name," said one. "An auspicious one," said another, as it came from a god. By naming our son in front of so many witnesses, my husband showed he would care for the boy. The naming bound the father to his son, to educating and bringing him up in the correct way.

We celebrated this with a great feast; a lamb was killed and the blood poured out to the gods. Many gifts were given to my son, as is the custom on the naming day. Toys, clothing, good luck charms and amulets were given to ward off the evil eye. It was a good day, indeed, and I held my head higher in the company of friends and family. Now I was a mother, a woman who had done what all expected of her.

Our son was a member of the family. He had been placed under the protection of our gods, welcomed by our relatives, and formally claimed by Isaeus. The only thing left was to prove that Apollodōrus was born of true citizens. This was important, for only legitimate sons could be citizens and take part in the important life of Athens. They could vote, hold office, and were the whole foundation of the polis (the city-state).[2]

At the end of the year, in the fall, Isaeus took our young son to the house of his brotherhood. All good families belonged to various brotherhoods, or phratries. At the brethren's house a priest sacrificed a sheep in honor of the

---

[2] This was so only for men. When a girl was declared legitimate, she could become the mother of other citizens. However, it did not entitle her to vote or take part in the political life of Athens.

child and prayed to the gods. Our son was then presented to all the brethren. They voted on whether Apollodōrus was a legitimate child. Of course, no man could question that! I was a true citizen, as was Isaeus; our son had to be declared legitimate and no bastard. Then his name was put in the register of the brotherhood. Forever, he was written down as a true citizen, a brother, and a member of the polis.

I cannot help but compare all the ceremonies to my weaving, and the thread to my son's life, spun out by the Fates. First, the shuttle is thrown across and the child becomes part of the immediate family; that happens during the fifth-day rite, the running around. Then comes the naming, and the child is woven more tightly into the piece of cloth growing on the loom; he becomes part of a wider kin group. Finally, the brethren and the polis make him part of themselves, and the thread is tightly pounded into place when the child's name is written down in the brotherhood's register. And what of the cloth that is growing on the loom? Why, that is my son's life as a boy and a man, a freeborn Athenian, member of the finest and noblest city known.

Birth in Hunting/Gathering Cultures

Chapter 3
TWO MOTHERS

Time: 1930
Place: The northwest mountains of Papuan New Guinea
Characters: An Arapesh clansman, his wife, and relatives

I was 8 when I was betrothed and sent to my husband's village. I was a shy and quiet girl, not given to loud and angry words like Temos, a girl of this village. I had left my father and brothers behind, left my mother and sisters for a new home.

The village was very like my old one, with round thatched huts on piles around a muddy clearing; coconut trees growing by the door; pigs and children running back and forth; and paths leading from the village like snakes' tails. Over the winding trails, the huts, and the green mountains hung the mist in white drifts, just as it had in my other village.

In time the strangeness left me. I cooked with my other mother, worked in the mountain gardens with my new sisters, and played with my new brothers. Manum, my husband-to-be, was as a brother to me then. He took my hand on the slippery paths and fed me taro and yams to make my body strong and healthy. In our village we say a husband is growing a wife when he does this, just as a man tends a plant in his garden.

As I changed over the next six years, I was careful to follow the taboos [1] guarding my growth. I did all that was

---

[1] These are rules forbidding certain acts in order to protect a person or people from the dangerous misuse of magic power.

needed to make my body into a woman's body. When my blood first came, I went to the women's huts outside the village and fasted longer than the other girls. After I came out of the menstrual hut, after the feasting and ceremonies, I never let myself be alone with my future husband. A man and woman must not make love until they are strong and full-grown; love too early can harm one's growth.

Some months after I first went to the women's huts, I felt I was ready for my husband. I was 15 years old, and Manum was a man of 20 years. He built a house for us and we lived together, waiting for a child. When the hot season came, I knew a child would grow inside. There had been no blood for many weeks, and it was time to tell Manum.

"Are you sure, Menala?" he asked after I told him. Then he touched his fine hairdo with the air of an important man and smiled. But Manum's smile faded as he looked gravely at me.

"Now the hard time begins, wife. For many weeks we will have to work together to make this child."

I nodded impatiently. Didn't I know how a child was formed? The father and mother must make love every night during the early weeks of pregnancy, as the man's seed joined with the mother's blood to form the baby.

"This is tiring work, Menala," my husband said to me many weeks later. He seemed to be getting thinner while I was getting rounder. "But," he added quickly, "I want this child, boy or girl, I want it."

I was calmed by that; a father must desire a child as much as the mother. How else can he have the strength to build the child inside the woman? And in the time after the birth, Manum's help and care would be as important as mine. For the husband grows yams and hunts animals to feed the child; he sleeps beside it each night that first year; and he helps clean the child and comfort it when it cries.

When I saw that my breasts had darkened and felt their swelling, I knew the difficult six weeks were over. I told Manum of the changes in my body, and he listened quietly.

"The child is finished then," he said. "Now he is like a round egg," Manum made a fist to show what the child looked like inside, "and he will rest in your body while we feed him."

"We must let him sleep, Manum," I said, and he signed his agreement. A husband and wife must not make love during the months ahead. It might jar the child awake, and that should not happen until the time of birth.

"When he wakes he will dive out like a fish," I said and laughed, thinking of that day. I hoped it would come soon, this birth, for the months of growing a child can be long and trying. There were many foods neither Manum nor I could eat, and places I could not go. Bandicoot was forbidden to me, the one that digs so deep in the ground. The child might be like him and never come out of my womb! And if I ate eels and frogs—the sudden, slippery ones—they would make the baby come too quickly, before he was ready. I would not touch sago or coconuts from sacred places, and must be careful never to walk deep in the bush where the marsalai lives [the supernatural guardian snake or lizard]. I also watched myself when preparing food and never cut anything in half—that would give me a girl. Manum and I had decided we wanted a son first.

One morning many months later, when the mist made all things the same, I felt the child turn over in me. It was the first time I'd felt it move,[2] and I put my hand over my taut skin to make certain. There—it moved again!

I shook Manum awake and he ran outside to get his sister, Una. I could hear her excited voice as she called to my other mother, Sagu, and my sister to come help. (My sister had also married a man of this village.) She had just borne a child herself and would tell me what to do throughout the birth. They came quickly and led me down the house ladder, over to the steep slope where the women's huts were. A birth could not take place within the village any more than a menstruating woman could stay in her regular house. Birth and women's blood are dangerous to men and can harm their yam gardens and their ability to hunt.

---

[2] The Arapesh believe a child doesn't move in the mother's body until the actual time of birth.

Down the wet path we went. Una holding one arm and my sister the other. The hut was not far off and I was glad to come to it, with the child loosening inside me.

On the hut's floor, my other mother spread fresh grass and moss and helped me crouch down. From the roof hung a woven rope, and my sister told me to hold onto it. I needed that support as I crouched, and it helped during the pains to pull hard on the rope. Una stood behind me so I could rest against her, while Sagu and my sister supported my knees.

That child was eager to come into the world, cold and rainy as it was! While I pulled on the rope, the baby put its hands over its head and dived out of my body into the waiting hands of Sagu.

She smiled when she saw the dark wrinkled baby was a boy. "A son!" she cried, "Manum will be happy." I knew he would be as glad as I was to welcome this son who was awake at last and outside my body.

Sagu gave the baby to my sister and stepped outside the birth hut. She called into the mist, "It is a son, a boy!"

From nearby came Manum's loud shout, "Clean the child!"

So a father tells whether he wants the child or not. If the baby is a girl and a man has two or three daughters already, he might call out, "Don't clean the child." Or if there is a famine in the village, he might say the same. Then the child is left in the bush to die.

But this was more a ritual for us now; there was no question that our baby would be kept, as he was our first. My hands trembled a little as I cut the cord with a bamboo sliver and made a knot in the piece left on the baby. My sister brought me warmed water in a coconut shell and we washed the baby together, cleaning off all traces of the birth.

He wailed as we washed him but stopped when we gently wiped him with grass. As soon as he was dry, I put him to my breast. While he sucked like a small, eager animal, the afterbirth came from my body. It felt to me as if the baby's sucking helped it to come out.

My other mother took the afterbirth and cord outside to put high in a tree, away from pigs, and then removed the grass and moss from the hut.

With all the birth fluids taken care of, the women led me back to the village. Once there, I could not go to my house; that would be too dangerous for the village. Instead, I went to a special, smaller hut, one with an earthen floor. There the dirt would absorb the danger and power that is on a woman who has just given birth.

I was glad to lie down on the grass bed the women had prepared for me, glad to lie quietly until my husband came. Soon Manum appeared in the doorway, trying to look old and wise but glowing like a boy who's just returned from his initiation.

"See," he said, walking carefully over to me, "I've brought water to wash the baby." He set down a filled coconut shell. "And," he held out some large leaves, "they will soften the net bag for the child. These are the special herbs," Manum said, as he sprinkled them about the floor, "that will keep evil ones away."

The smell of those magic plants filled the small room and made me feel safe.

Manum lay down near me, looking eagerly at the baby between us. I was happy to have my husband here at last, to share this birth with him. The child came from my womb, but he also came from Manum's body. My husband was as much a part of the birth as I was.

Manum takes up the narration:

It was good to lie down beside my wife and small child, to rest together. A husband is also tired by the work of bearing a child. Those hard weeks so long ago, when I had helped build the child inside Menala, had aged me. Now, in the special hut, I would stay beside the baby for five days, helping to grow him and make him strong. That time is like a birth, and the life-soul that lives like a butterfly under a child's bones is then as much the father's as the mother's. So we say of a man when he is in the small hut with his wife and new one, "He is in bed having a baby." [3]

I knew husbands must give advice to their wives during this time; that is the custom of the mountain people and one my father had prepared me for. He spoke to me of the ways of caring for and growing the child. I now told Menala, "Move the baby closer to my chest." There he would be warmer and the cold mists could not reach him.

So we spent that afternoon and evening lying next to the baby, resting from our long labor and holding the child. For the first day only, we did not eat, smoke, or drink water. Such things might harm the new one. Through that day, as would be so for the next five days, I could not scratch myself with my hand, but must use a stick. I could not eat with my fingers, but must use a spoon. Work was forbidden to me, as was hunting and tending my yam garden. Birth-time is dangerous to a man when he is so close to it in the special hut. He must act carefully to keep the danger of the birthblood from his mouth, his garden, and the sacred places of the bush.

The next morning my brothers' wives came to help with the child, bringing with them the magic things to make the boy grow strong and healthy. Kumati, one of the wives, brought a long stick with the bark taken off. Without the bark, it could better absorb magic power.

I looked outside the hut and called in some of the healthiest children playing outside. While they crowded eagerly around the baby, I held the peeled stick in my hand and rubbed it over each child's back, over the fine black skin and the strong bones inside. That rod was like a bit of dry earth soaking up the day's rain; it would take into itself all the goodness in those children's backs. Then I took the stick and rubbed it over our baby's back, chanting this charm:

---

[3] Margaret Mead, "The Mountain-Dwelling Arapesh," *Sex and Temperament in Three Primitive Societies* (New York: William Morrow & Co., 1935), p. 33.

> *"I give you the small bones of the back,*
> *one from a pig,*
> *one from a snake,*
> *one from a human being,*
> *one from a tree-snake,*
> *one from a python,*
> *one from a viper,*
> *and one from a child."* [4]

Afterward, I broke the stick into small pieces and hid them in the hut. This would protect our son's back from being hurt if I stepped on a stick outside.

Before I could take up my old life again, and before Menala and I could return to our house, I had to be cleansed of the close contact with my wife, still dangerous from birth and its blood. This purifying ceremony came at the end of the five days in the hut. To direct it, I chose Gerud, an older man of the village who had borne many children.

He led me away from the dark hut and down to a pool outside the village. Magic herbs had been put in the pool, and I drank of the clear water, cleansing my mouth. Gerud told me to walk into the water and wash my body. In the cold pool I felt all the danger of my days in the hut taken from by body. Now I could work again, could go to my yam gardens, could walk in the bush. On my forehead Gerud put a white spot, which marked me as a true father, one who had given birth to a healthy child.

Back in the small shelter, Menala and I held a feast to celebrate the return to our everyday lives. All our close relatives in the village came to see the baby and share our food. There was a burst of excited talk in the doorway and Una came in, followed by my brothers and their wives, my mother and father, and Menala's sister. Our baby made them laugh by waving his arms and suddenly falling asleep.

[4] Ibid., p. 34.

"Ah, he's a smart one, that child," said one brother.

"And look at his nose, just like his father's," Una said.

The rest tried to find out if the baby looked more like Menala or me; that is how you know where the child's soul comes from—the mother's or father's line. It was still too early to tell, and my mother scolded us when she said. "Don't hurry the child! There will be time enough before we know who he is like."

My mother was right. You could not make a child grow faster than he would, and it would be wrong to hurry him.

The feast that day was a good one, and an important one. The nuts and tobacco we gave our visitors were like threads binding them to me and to Menala. The men would give special help to me when I needed it, in building a house or in gardening, and the women would help Menala when she needed them.

At last we returned to our big house, and my wife climbed swiftly up the house ladder. The baby bumped gently against her back, and if you did not look closely, you could hardly see him curled up inside her net bag. Menala sighed and sat down on the floor, and I crouched beside her. We were both happy to be back, even though we knew we must live carefully with our newborn.

Here, in our own house, I would stay by my son and wife each night until the child could walk. How else can the child grow unless the father is with him every night? And all through the months until the child walked, I would not make love with Menala. That would harm the baby's growth; we must wait until the child was bigger and stronger.

The boy was a delight to me. I know some fathers are restless and wish to leave on trading journeys or visit other villages, but I was content to follow our custom and stay near the child.

Each day I held him and played with him, waiting for the day he would first laugh. At last it came, on a hot misty morning. I was tickling the baby's feet when he looked up at me and laughed.

"Menala, Menala!" I called out. "Did you hear him? He laughed!" and she came quickly to see.

"He is ready for his name now," she said.

Among our people, a child is never named until he first laughs in his father's face. I called our son Maigi, after a cousin from my father's clan. It was a fine name, and I was glad to call him something other than "little one" or "baby."

That night as Menala and I sat around the fire, talking softly and looking at Maigi asleep in my lap, I thought how good it was to have a son. I would love my daughters too, when they came, but a daughter is not with you for long. As Menala said to me, "He'll stay with us and won't leave for other villages to be married, as our daughters will."

"A son is good for his parents' old age," I agreed.

I thought of the years ahead, how Menala and I would care for the boy and help him grow. All that we did would be for Maigi, to make his bones strong and his body healthy. Then, one day, after his pubic hair came in, he would be ready to join the sacred men's cult and leave childhood behind. The child had come from my wife's body, but only the men of our clan can give birth to men. This is our sacred knowledge, how boys are changed into men, and my wife and other women knew nothing of it. Such knowledge might harm their ability to bear children.

One day our son would walk with other boys his age into the sacred walled area at the edge of the village. There, we kept the boys away from women for three months. During that time, we fed the younger ones special foods to make them grow and beat them with stinging nettles to make them strong. The older men cut the boys on their arms, for that blood-letting helps cleanse them. Then the clansmen take their own blood and mix it with coconut milk to feed to the younger ones; just so did the boys receive blood and milk from their mothers' bodies so long ago. This rite grows the boys into men, as they now have men's blood in them as well as women's. All the ceremonies in the sacred area are to change boys into full members of the clan—strong ones who can garden, hunt, and father children.

After the three months in the initiation place—and how good that time is, with singing, feasting, and learning the secrets of the Tamberan [5]—the changed ones come out of the walled circle, just as children are born from their mothers' bodies. Now the boys are men, born of their clansmen's blood and the sacred Tamberan. Round and shining, Maigi would return to the village, ready to start his life as a grown person. In time, he would marry and begin the glad work of bearing children. Our son would become a man whose life would be to grow others, as we had for so long and so lovingly grown him.

---

[5] The sacred guardian of the men's cult, seen as an enormous man who brings health and fertility to the tribe.

Chapter 4
THAT MY HOOD BE FULL

> Time: 1918
> Place: Thule, Greenland
> Characters: A Polar Eskimo family

They were hurrying to reach the tiny settlement before the gale struck. Only a day's journey away, they were returning from a trip to pick up meat caches for the month of no sun (December). All day a sharp, biting wind blew against the travelers, frosting their eyelashes and turning the skin on their noses white from frostbite. On top of the sledge sat a woman, Ivalu, and her 3-year-old son, asleep. Sometimes she slept as her husband, Samik, drove between the stanchions. But when the sled hit rough ice or had to go uphill, she quickly jumped off and ran beside it.

A white man, a foreigner, might not know the woman was pregnant. Here, in the far North, the bulky winter furs of the Polar Eskimos disguised the full body of Ivalu. But she and her husband knew the birth would come soon. That morning, on the trail, Ivalu had felt a few twinges, not enough to signal the birth, just a reminder: "It will happen soon; hurry, hurry home."

She'd told Samik that morning, with the characteristic understatement of an Eskimo, "It is not impossible that a baby may be born today." Samik had hardly shown surprise as he looked at his wife and son on top of the sled. "One must hurry, then," was all he said, and he whipped up his dogs, letting each one feel the tip of the lash.

Over the hard-packed snow they drove, the dogs yapping excitedly, their tails standing straight up. Throughout the afternoon, Ivalu either rode on top of the sled or ran beside it to warm her feet. Even as her pains started, she continued to trot alongside.

The only thing Ivalu said to her husband was, "One has a stomachache," as she climbed back onto the sled to rest.

Samik's thoughts raced along with his dogs: Should he stop now and build an igloo? Did they have time to reach the village and the warm sod hut that awaited them?

"Is it possible you might wait until we get home?" Samik asked his wife. It would not be accurate to say he was worried; if she could not travel all the way back they'd stop and build a snow shelter where the child could be born. He would adjust to whatever happened, saying, "We will stop here," or "Home is just ahead."

Ivalu listened inside herself, trying to find an answer. Could she wait? How far along was her labor? It was her third child, after all (her first, a son named Odark, was at home with his grandmother), and she knew her labor would be short, not more than three or four hours of the white man's time. But her pains had started only a little way back. She signed to her husband that he should continue and said, "One can wait."

Samik whipped up the dogs again, and they strained against their harness. Racing through the driving wind and the dark, Samik relied on the dogs' sense of direction to take them home, and on his own intimate knowledge of each bump and ridge in the white landscape.

Later, as Ivalu held her son, swaying with the sled's motion and straining her eyes ahead for a pinpoint of light, she suddenly sat up higher. "Samik, one sees a light! There's a house ahead!"

The dogs announced their arrival, barking and snarling at each other as they came to a stop. People hurried out of the sod huts to welcome the travelers and help them unload. Samik's mother, Mequ, took her grandson off the sledge, while Samik gently helped his wife to the ground. Normally, she'd jump off first and run into the house, calling out greetings. But now she was glad of his strength and let herself be led to the tunnel entrance where she dropped to her knees and crawled inside. Samik had already told Mequ what was happening, and she hurried to remove Ivalu's outer fur parka and beat the snow from it. Then she drew off Ivalu's long sealskin boots and her bearskin pants. That done, she took her grandson, Manik, to the sleeping platform at the back of the room. There he would be out of the way. The boy was tired from his long journey and soon put his head in his grandmother's lap to sleep.

Samik called a greeting to his older son, who was already on the platform, curled in his fur bag. But the man had no time to talk with his son, and as Odark looked on, wide-eyed, Samik pulled bundles from the walls into the center of the floor. Quickly, he put two rolls of hides near each other, making an armrest for Ivalu. Next, he scraped a shallow hole in the earthen floor and lined it with a caribou skin.

Ivalu knelt down between the bundles and rested her arms on them. They supported her on the side, and she sighed with relief to be here at last. "It will happen soon," she told her husband, who knelt behind her. Ivalu leaned back, letting her weight rest against him. Samik and Ivalu had already had two children, and he knew what to do. Putting his arms around his wife's abdomen, he began to press down firmly on the unborn baby. Ivalu felt the child kick once, a small protest from the one inside. Then the descent began, and she could feel the baby being pushed out of her body by Samik. The pressure of the child against the birth-opening forced her legs wider apart. In a rush, like a tiny, slippery seal, the baby slid out onto the caribou skin below. It cried once, twice, and then was still.

Samik looked down at the tiny red figure lying in the hole. "*Ee-ee,* it's a girl! Is she not lovable?"

Ivalu was concentrating on the rest of the birth and could hardly let herself be relieved at her husband's delight. For the father can decide whether a girl will be kept or killed so the wife can get pregnant again to bear, hopefully, a boy. Sons support their parents in their old age and are more desirable than girls. But they had two sons already, and the hunting had been good this year—the girl would live.

Samik looked beneath Ivalu to see how things were progressing. He went up to his wife's head and spoke softly to her. "Try pushing a little. It hasn't come yet."

Ivalu strained her body, but the afterbirth was not ready to come out. Samik tried calling to it: "Come out bad afterbirth! Come out now!"

As he continued to call to the afterbirth to be born, scolding it for being so slow, the placenta finally was expelled.

Quickly, Ivalu turned around on her knees to face the child. Samik handed her the *ulo*, the curved steel knife used for scraping skins, and Ivalu cut the umbilical cord. In the old days, before white men came to Greenland with their trading stations, she would have bitten through the navel cord or cut it with a stone knife. Now she knotted a sinew around the cut cord to stop the bleeding.

She picked up the small, quiet girl, wiped her dry with a foxskin, and put the child to her breast. The baby was soft and warm against her own naked skin, and though the hut was heated with blubber lamps, Ivalu wrapped the baby in a piece of fur. For a moment, the small head wavered over the breast. Then she found the nipple and began to suck noisily, with surprising strength.

"*Ee-ee,* she's a quick one!" the father said, smiling at his wife.

"*Vaaa,*" she murmured, a sign of affectionate approval.

Samik wrapped the afterbirth in the caribou hide and stood up to take it outside. He could not bury the bundle in the frozen ground, but just left it beyond the settlement, knowing the foxes would find it.

Inside the hut, Ivalu sat happily nursing the child while her mother-in-law looked on. Mequ talked softly to herself about the children she had borne, the ones who had died, and others she had had to kill during times of famine.

"Five big boys," she murmured to no one in particular,

puffing on a cigarette. "And three girls—only one could live."

Samik turned his mother's attention away from the past to the present by asking, "What should we name the new one, eh? Perhaps one might call in the *Angakok* [shaman] to discover the child's name."

At that moment, the baby lost her mother's nipple and began to wail.

"She's crying for her name," Ivalu said, with a smile.

"Let an old one see," Mequ said, and came over to peer at the new one. Ivalu turned her body so the grandmother could see the baby's face.

"Eh," Mequ said. "Her nose is as fine and small as my own mother's. No one in the village had such a beautiful flat nose as Navarana did. Perhaps my mother has been reborn in this one." She thought some more and then said definitely, "Navarana is alive again; their faces are the same."

"Navarana it is," the father said, pleased that such a good name had been found. He knew his grandmother had been a skilled sewer, something much desired in an Eskimo woman. Along with her name, the grandmother's sewing ability and beauty were also given to the baby. Now she was a complete human being, as all people are made of three things: a body, a soul, and a name. To protect the child from evil spirits that roamed outside in the howling wind, Samik gave his daughter three other names—Atitak, Iva, and Kullabak. For a name is magic, almost a soul in itself.

Mequ went over to the back of the hut and rummaged around in a pile of her belongings. She came back and sat beside Ivalu.

"Here, daughter, to help bring her sons." Mequ held out a small, twisted thing.

"Thank you, mother," Ivalu said. "A poor woman does not deserve such a fine gift," and she took up the dried dovekie's foot. Tied by a sinew, it would become an amulet for her daughter to wear. Because dovekies have such large eggs, the Eskimos believed a girl who wore this dried bird's foot would then bear large sons.

Now that the baby had nursed, Ivalu took her over to her oldest boy, Odark, who was lying on the sleeping platform. He had tried to stay awake for the birth, but was too tired to watch the whole process. He had seen his mother kneeling on the floor, heard a few soft comments, and then gone back to sleep.

"Look at the new one," Ivalu said.

Odark stretched, yawned, and touched the nose of the tiny red baby.

"A little sister, eh? I can teach her how to drive dogs, and she can play with me in the snow."

"*Ee-ee,* wait until she learns to walk first!" Ivalu laughed.

Then she took the baby to her youngest son, Manik, who had to be shaken from sleep. He woke to find himself no longer king, no more the only child with exclusive right to his mother's breasts. Though he was 3 years old, he still nursed regularly.

"Look at your new sister." Ivalu held up the baby.

Manik didn't say anything, but just wrinkled his nose in the Eskimo gesture meaning, "No."

Ivalu smiled and rubbed his nose affectionately with hers. "You are still loved, great big son. Come, have tea."

The grandmother handed around cups of the hot steaming liquid, which they all drank, sitting on the platform. In time, they would lie down together, each in his or her place. The baby would sleep between Ivalu and Samik, while the youngest boy would have to move to a new place. From now on, he would sleep between his father and his older brother.

Ivalu sipped her tea, thinking of tomorrow and the excitement it would bring. Samik would tell everyone in the small settlement of the birth, and visitors would come throughout the day to see the baby and talk. The tiny girl would be passed from hand to hand, nuzzled, petted, and cooed over. That night, someone might have a celebration with dancing and music in one of the new wooden houses built by the Danish traders. Then she would pop her baby into her *amaut,* the pouch-like section of her parka, and go to the party. She would feel the naked baby warm against her back and could sing to herself:

> *"It's my big baby*
> *That I feel in my hood—*
> *Oh how heavy she is!*
> *Ya ya! Ya ya!*
>
> *"When I turn*
> *She smiles at me, my little one,*
> *Oh how heavy she is!*
> *Ya ya! Ya ya!*
>
> *"How sweet she is when she smiles*
> *With her mouth like a little seal's.*
> *Ah, I like my baby to be heavy*
> *And my hood to be full."* [1]

---

[1] Adapted from Jean Malaurie, *The Last Kings of Thule,* trans. by Gwendolen Freeman (New York: Thomas Y. Crowell Company, 1956), p. 100.

Birth in an Agricultural Tribe

Chapter 5
THE MIDDLE PLACE

Time: 1896
Place: The Zuñi Pueblo, western New Mexico
Characters: A Zuñi Indian family

When the first people searched for a home, according to Zuñi legend, they came to a dry, reddish land where the sun and the stars and the moon kept watch. There, a shallow river ran across the plain and a huge tableland rose beyond. In that place, which they called the Middle of the World, the first Zuñis built their pueblo.

Through the centuries, the Zuñi Indians lived in the Middle Place. They survived the Spaniards with their cruel mouths and the beasts that ran beneath their legs. They outlasted the white strangers with double tongues, who told them about a terrible place of burning fire under the earth. Those men were confused and not to be noticed, only pitied as children who have not yet reached the age of reason.

In the pueblo that rose like a storied mesa from the red earth, a woman named We' wha was with child, It had been a bad year for children and crops, and We' wha was glad of the baby inside. A birth was always welcome, especially now with the whites on the move and the Navahos, their ancient enemies, ready to raid their village. A new child would add its life to the pueblo, would help the Zuñis grow as their corn flourished in the dry land.

We' wha felt a quiet strength and serenity about her child. She had already borne one, a boy, two years ago. Her body was not frail, like a white woman's, but was short and broad—made for bearing children. She was sure this birth would be a safe one, for had she not seen Cha' kwena (the guardian of childbirth) at the great winter festival? During that dark time, when the Zuñis invited the rain gods into their homes, the guardian of childbirth came to their village and danced majestically in the square. All pregnant women hurried to look at her, believing they would then be given a safe delivery.

After the winter sun returned in strength to the village, We' wha knew it was time to go to Mother rock, the sacred place visited by pregnant Zuñi women. She and her husband wanted a girl this time, and certain acts and sacred words could bring them a female child.

Outside the village, the great mesa rose and shone a dull copper red in the late afternoon light. At the foot of Mother rock was an overhang, covered with the signs for a woman's vulva. There, We' wha, her husband, and her sister gathered. The pregnant woman scraped some rock dust from the overhang and put it in a tiny vase. This she later placed in a hole in Mother rock. All three prayed that a girl would be born to We' wha, and that the child would be beautiful, kind, a good potter, and a skilled weaver. The husband and wife remembered their hearts must be single and pure if their prayers were to be answered. Fixing their thoughts on the unborn child, they returned to the pueblo, now earth-colored in the dusk. Another step had been taken on the road that led to birth, another rite completed that would make the child healthy and good.

The rest of We' wha's pregnancy went as smoothly and placidly as the Zuñi river that ran by the pueblo. Only once did she fear for her child, when a bitter woman without children sat next to her. They were on the flat roof of the house, grinding corn with a stone, when We' wha remembered the tales told about the serpent-tongued woman. For witches have "double tongues and paired thoughts"[1] and can harm the child inside the mother. We' wha found an excuse and hurriedly left to go inside. It would be madness to stay next to a woman suspected of witchcraft. Could she not cast worms into a mother's womb that would then devour the baby?

During the next week, We' wha carefully felt her belly each morning and listened inside herself for the sounds of gnawing. She told no one, not even her husband, afraid that talking of the evil might make it real. Only after she was sure no harm had been done did she go about the village again. Her face no longer looked like the winter sky over the desert and became again the serene face of a Zuñi woman who carries a child.

In late spring, when the harsh winds drove the desert before them, We' wha's husband left for his fields. It was time to plant corn, and he hoped he could till and finish planting before his child was born.

The Zuñi woman said little when he walked away and only watched his figure growing smaller and smaller in the distance until he became part of the red and yellow sand.

A few days after he left, on a gray, windy morning, We' wha felt her first pains. She hardly let herself wish her husband home; all her attention must now be fixed on the coming birth. It was not as if she were alone. Living in her mother's house, she was surrounded by a warm and caring family.

Holding her hand to her body, We' wha did not hurry to look for her mother or shout for her sisters. Quietly, she went inside, took her seat on the wall ledge, and signed to her mother that the pains had started.

"My daughter!" The old woman was more excited than We' wha. "Let me make a bed for you at this end of the room."

Smiling and bustling with the joy of this, her third grandchild, K' iawu gathered up sheepskins from the

[1] Frank Hamilton Cushing. *Zuñi Folk Tales* (New York: The Knickerbocker Press, 1901). p. 14.

storeroom and brought them into the main living room. She spread them on the floor, making a soft, warm bed for her daughter.

"Here, We' wha," said the older woman, as she helped the young one off the sitting ledge and onto the sheepskins.

One of her sisters took We' wha's little boy and her own infant into a corner of the room. There, during the labor and birth, she would stay with the children and keep them quiet.

Almost humming with excitement, K' iawu went off to find the old women of the family and bring them back to help with the birth. In a few minutes, We' wha's two grandmothers entered the low room and greeted the pregnant woman.

"My daughter, how is it with you?"

"My mothers, it is well."

One had brought juniper wood with her and proceeded to build up the fire and boil water for tea in a clay pot. When the water was ready, she put in the juniper twigs and berries to let them brew. Then the grandmother handed a cup of this hot tea to We' wha.

The pregnant woman sat up to take the healing liquid and cradled the cup in her hands. The heat felt good, and she breathed deeply of the fragrant steam. From past experience, We' wha knew juniper tea helped during labor. It would relax her body and keep her limbs from knotting during the hard time ahead.

For the next two hours, We' wha alternately sipped tea and lay back on her sheepskin bed. When the pains came, she pushed her feet hard against the sitting ledge. Occasionally, when her legs began to cramp, she got up and walked slowly around the room. No sound escaped her; there were no groans or cries for sympathy. We' wha just pressed her lips together and thought of the proper behavior for Zuñi women. They did not cry out, like white women, or make much of their labor. They simply went through it and kept silent, as they had been taught.

Later, around dusk, one grandmother decided it was time to call in a doctress. We' wha had been in labor for ten hours now, and there was nothing to show for it. Another daughter of the house was sent off to find a doctress, carrying the proper presents for her services.

The daughter returned with two women, who came into the living room and sat down by We' wha. One felt carefully over the unborn child, while the other arranged the laboring woman's pillow and blanket.

The older doctress said, "My sisters, this one is slow for a second birth."

To speed up the delivery, both women put their hands on We' wha's abdomen and began to knead it vigorously. Although We' wha gritted her teeth, a moan escaped her as the strong hands worked over her body. She wanted to draw her knees up and cry out, "Stop, enough!" But she waited a little, and the kneading had an effect. Suddenly she felt something let go and her legs were wet.[2]

One doctress lifted the blanket and examined her patient.

"*Hoya* [thanks], sister, this is helping her," and she pointed to the fluid. In their experience, they knew the baby often followed soon after.

The older doctress said, "Turn over on your side, my daughter, and we will bring the baby out."

We' wha turned over and held onto the belt of the doctress before her. Behind, the older woman put her hands on We' wha's back and pressed hard, trying to push the baby out of the mother.

To the pregnant woman, the pushing was a relief. Her pains were cutting now, like the arrows of the warrior gods, and that pressure on her back lessened some of the pain. Just to feel the child would come was a help.

The women of the family groaned in sympathy with We' wha, and some wept. If their sister could not show her emotion, the family could, and they gave for her the sighs and moans of childbirth.

In the adjoining room, the men of the family waited anxiously. Smoking and talking in low voices were We'

---

[2] The amniotic sac (or bag of waters) had broken.

wha's unmarried brother, her uncle, her father and her grandfather. They concentrated on the coming birth, believing that their thoughts would help the child be born.

But the older doctress was not satisfied with her patient's progress. She decided to give that stubborn baby an extra push. The doctress pinched We' wha's nostrils together and blew into her mouth. Two or three times, the woman tried to "blow" the child out of the mother's body.

Each time We' wha coughed and had to sit up to catch her breath again. Yet she would endure anything to help her baby be born.

The doctresses talked together about the delayed birth; should they send for the priests of the Great Fire brotherhood? The wise ones would pray to the beast gods for a speedy delivery, and the sacred songs of power would bring the child out.

While they were discussing the proper gifts to send to the priests, We' wha grabbed onto one woman's belt and began to give birth to her child. Hurriedly, the older doctress lifted the blanket above We' wha's knees and turned her on her back. Sitting on the wall ledge and positioning herself between the laboring woman's knees, the doctress held out her hands. At the same time, the two grandmothers helped to steady We' wha's legs. As soon as the dark head of the baby appeared, the doctress gently put her hands on either side of the infant's head. Shaking it slightly, she slowly pulled the baby toward her. As she pulled, the other woman kneaded We' wha's stomach.

Blue as a winter shadow, the baby slid out of We' wha's body.[3] A broad smile creased the old one's face as she said, "My sisters, another daughter for you!" She held up the baby girl. The other doctress cut the navel cord with a knife and pressed it to stop the bleeding. Then she wrapped a thick cotton string around the cord.

For the first time, We' wha began to cry. She wanted to hold the child, to number all its fingers, to see if it was

---

[3] Babies are blue at birth and become red shortly after they begin to breathe.

alive. But she was not through with the birthing. One doctress kept kneading her abdomen until the afterbirth was delivered. The grandmother quickly put it in a bowl and took it outside to the river that gleamed in the moonlight. With prayers that We' wha would have many more healthy children, the grandmother let the afterbirth fall into the river, and hurried back to the pueblo.

Inside, the fire kept the chill night air from the family. The initial activity over, they congratulated We' wha on her baby girl and talked quietly among themselves. Carefully and intently, the family watched the attempts of the doctresses to bring a cry or wail from the baby. For the infant was slow to respond to the touch and sounds of the women around her.

The two doctresses and grandmothers continually stroked and tickled the child to make her move and respond. One tickled the infant's feet, while another blew gently into her mouth. The grandmother rubbed the baby's face and tapped her nose. The baby's chest was massaged and her arms moved up and down. Blankets warmed by the fire were kept wrapped around the child.

Then a high thin wail rewarded them, and the baby feebly moved one hand. It was as if no other child had ever been born before.

"My sisters, look at her eyes!"

"My daughter, look, her foot is moving!"

"Little one, little one," the women murmured, as they continued to stroke and blow on the baby. Then the child was held up for all to see, like a small talisman, proof that life is stronger than death. Carefully, as if to wrap the newly won life within the child, the baby was enfolded in another small blanket and held on the doctress's lap.

Now that We' wha was certain her child would live, she rose from her bed and took a heated stone from the ashes. Wrapping it in her belt, she tied it around her stomach and felt the welcome heat seep into her sore body. She sat by the fire and drank a cup of steaming juniper tea, its heat filling her inside.

The two grandmothers cleaned We' wha's bed, piling

sand on the sheepskin to absorb the birth fluids. The sand was swept up and taken outside.

We' wha's father and mother brought in clean, wet sand and put it on the floor. One doctress took two heated flat stones, and putting half of the pile to one side, she rubbed the sand between the warm stones. Again and again, she worked the sand until it was dry and completely heated. She scooped out two places in the sand bed—one for the baby's head, and one for her body. Over the bed she spread a warmed cloth. The other doctress put sacred cornmeal at the head of the mound and prayed to the Master of Life and The Sun Father that the child would be strong and long-lived. A line of sacred meal was sprinkled from east to west across the bed, a sign for the straight path of life the girl must walk to win the gods' blessings. After the prayers, the infant was laid on the sand bed and an ear of corn put by her side. The corn represented the well-being of the Zuñi, and would help bring health and fertility to the baby girl.

We' wha then had a sand bed prepared for her, with hot stones heating and drying the sand. Near the mound, K'iawu put down bowls of steaming mutton soup, hot bread, and cornmeal mush. The tired new mother sat down on her comforting bed and ate gladly of the food, with the rest of the family joining in the meal.

After the hard birth, after her pain, We' wha was wrapped in warmth, as her child had been. Her family around her, a part of warm mother earth beneath her, We' wha slept for a time.

Outside the pueblo, the sky changed from black to gray, to a dusky red with streaks of yellow. The older doctress, who had not slept, noticed the golden light and nodded to the women of the family. With the rays of their Sun Father entering the room, it was time to bathe the child. One grandmother brought a bowl of warm water and a basket filled with ashes. Taking the child onto her lap, the older doctress filled her mouth with water and spit it out over the baby's face. After washing the head, the doctress rubbed ashes into the infant's face. That was to purify the child for her first sight of the Sun Father, and also to keep hair from growing on her.

Then the doctress unwrapped the tiny girl and washed her entire body, again rubbing ashes into the skin. A warmed blanket was wrapped around the now smudged baby. A new sand bed was prepared and heated, and the child laid upon it.

We' wha watched the ritual bathing and thought how beautiful her child was, even covered with ashes. Her dark eyes were lively, and her hands curled and uncurled.

Now it was We' wha's turn to be bathed and cleansed. Her mother had brewed root tea, and the doctress told We' wha to lie down on the bed. Cupping some root tea in her hand, the woman bathed We' wha's vulva and the surrounding area, soothing the sore flesh. Then the doctress sprinkled a medicinal powdered root over the washed skin. After the healing bath, the doctress kneaded We' wha's abdomen. That would help her body return to its normal size and would also expel the birth fluids. Like all Zuñi women who have just delivered, We' wha continued to drink hot juniper tea. It would stop the birth fluids in three or four days, sooner than any white man's tea or medicine.

Though We' wha tried to nurse her baby in the following days, her milk did not come in. But the child would not go hungry, for We' wha's sister had a suckling baby. She would nurse the child until the mother's milk appeared.

On the sixth day after the birth, We' wha's baby was presented to the Zuñi gods. A line of sacred meal was sprinkled from the house to the door, and the older doctress carried the child in her arms to see the Sun Father. Facing east, she prayed for the health and long life of the child:

> "*May your road be fulfilled*
> *Reaching to the road of your Sun Father* . . ."[4]

---

[4] Ruth L. Bunzel, "Introduction to Zuñi Ceremonialism," Annual Report o. the Bureau of American Ethnology, no. 47 (Washington D.C.: Government Printing Office, 1932), p. 636.

With dark curious eyes, the infant looked on the rising sun. Those same eyes continued to look around her as she was carried back into the pueblo. There both mother and child were washed with froth made from beaten yucca plants. This finally cleansed and purified them after the birth. During the washing, the doctress asked that all blessings of the gods be given to this child, this little one who was just starting on the path of life.

Soon, the child would be strapped to the beautiful cradle her grandfather was making. And sooner still, she would be held in the arms of another warm, loving person—her father, who was hurrying home from his corn fields to see his newborn daughter.

Birth in Urban Cultures

Chapter 6
MY THOUSAND OUNCES OF GOLD

Time: 1860
Place: Fuchau, China
Characters: A Chinese merchant's family

Her eyes were like black pebbles, and I hated her from the moment she came to my husband's house. She was pretty and young, all the things I was not. But it was my husband's desire to take her into his house, and I could do nothing. I was carrying his child, and he could no longer come to me at night. For the husband and wife must stay apart if impure influences are to be kept from the baby growing inside. My most honorable husband moved his concubine into her own room in the women's apartments. And I? I "ate vinegar," as other wives have before me.

Such is the will of heaven, and I must accept it, as women accept all things that come to them in this life. Yet under my heart I had a joy that almost made up for the pebble-eyed whore—a baby.

I had done much for this child, going often to the temple of Mother [the goddess of childbirth] and burning incense and candles before her image. At home, before her altar, I prayed daily for a son to rescue me from dishonor in my husband's house, to save me from a mother-in-law who would not stop scolding. What can I say of that one, except her mouth is as wide as the mouth of hell, and the sounds that come from it are like the cries of demons?

In my desire for a son, I even went to the fortune-teller who sees into the future. She looked at my flower-tree in the other world and told me how it grew. In that unseen world, each woman has a tree. On it red flowers (girls) may grow, or white flowers (boys) may bloom. If there are both red and white blossoms, the woman will bear boys and girls. Sometimes the tree is diseased or without flowers; I feared mine was like that. But the gracious fortune-teller said my tree had both white and red flowers on it, and that the tree was healthy and strong.

I came home from her house with happiness in my heart. The curse of barrenness was not on me. I would have a child, and I prayed it would be a son. Only a boy can offer incense and food to the memory of his parents; only a son can sweep their graves clean.

And if I could not bear a son, then I—Ling, daughter of a scholar and poet—could be divorced and put away. That is why I kept my anger about the black-eyed whore to myself. How could she hurt me, now that I carried my husband's child? Even she, with her skin like white silk and her tiny petal feet, could not take my worthy husband from me.

I grew fat like the moon in the season of silkworms. And as moths are drawn to the moon, so the women of our house fluttered around me. Even my bronze-tongued mother-in-law was careful of me during that time. What could she do for "her Ling?" Did I desire volumes of fine poetry or the blind storyteller down the street? I said "yes" to all her suggestions and basked in the rare attention. I listened to beautiful poetry and stories; delicate pictures were hung in my room, and my clothes were of brightly colored silk. All these things would create good influences around the baby. No bad words could reach my ears, no ugly sights offend me, no bad food be given to me.

My husband's mother, Li, even had me take an old fish net along when I went out in my sedan chair. That evil-smelling thing was draped over the sedan door to frighten away demons and bad spirits. Because fish nets resemble the demon-catching nets of the priest, they scare away the harmful ones. So my mother-in-law told me.

During the fifth month of my pregnancy, we held the

special ceremony to thank Mother. What good foods we put out for her on the table lit with candles! We burned the best incense and the shiniest mock-money that could be found. Mother is always pleased by such gifts. The priest asked the goddess for her continued protection during my pregnancy, and for an easy delivery at the end.

As silkworms spin their webs, my time closed in on me. The eighth month came, and Li engaged the most skillful midwife in all Fuchau. Nothing would go wrong with her grandson's birth, if she could prevent it! It was Li who decided to hold the rite to placate the demons of childbirth. People fear that at the time of a confinement, two evil females rise from hell to torture and even kill the laboring woman. To drive them away, we put out plates of food and burned incense and mock-money.

When the harvest moon hung low and orange in the black sky, my pains came. At first they were no worse than a backache. I was led away by Li, who put me to bed and piled warm quilts around me. Leaving my old nurse, she and the midwife went to pray before the house image of Mother. I knew they were asking the goddess for a fast and easy delivery. Then they would worship the ancestors, asking the help of all good spirits.

In bed, with the curtains drawn, I was suddenly lonely and afraid. Would I die? I was not a young woman, and I had heard of others, old as I, dying in childbirth. I did not wholly believe in demons, as Li did, but I shivered and thought of the Bloody Lake in hell. There, women who die in childbirth go to a comfortless, grim end.

I cried out to my old nurse: "Hsin Nai-nai? Are you still there? Talk with me, tell me stories, anything to make this time pass!"

Her kind, wrinkled face poked through the bed curtains and she sat beside me. Patting my shaking hands with her firm ones, she then smoothed my hair back.

"There now, did I ever tell you how the moon rabbit fell in love with the sun?" Her calm voice went on, telling the loved and known story to her mistress, who suddenly felt 6 years old again and afraid.

I should have saved my fear for later, saved my strength.

My labor went on and on; through that night, through sunset of the next day. In the dim, hazy world I lived in, I knew people were gathering outside my bed. A Taoist priest came and muttered prayers in my ear. I wanted to shout to him, "Speak to that one down there; the one who refuses to come out! Don't prattle to me!" He only waved some charms written on yellow paper, burned one and mixed it with water. This I had to drink, to make the child come.

It did not. More hours had gone by when I heard the sounds of people in the room. Li drew open the bed curtains and told me to look at the doorway. There were the puppeteers with their gay, bright puppets. For the first time in many hours, my heart lifted. One of the puppets was an image of Mother, while the others were her helpers. They danced and turned in the doorway, and it almost seemed the goddess was there. Then, since I was old for a first birth and my labor was long, the puppeteer came and put the image of Mother on my stomach. Three times the tiny goddess moved swiftly down to the birth-opening. So the child should move, as quickly and as easily.

That small face with the calm smile and dark eyes soothed me. With one part, I knew it was only a puppet. But the other part welcomed Mother to my bed and prayed for the child's descent.

Then I was alone again. Like a sudden leaf storm, my visitors disappeared and only the midwife and old nurse remained.

With a voice more cheerful than she looked, the midwife said, "Now he'll come, mistress. I've never seen that to fail once. Mother always brings the child out."

Was it the power of her words or the puppet that changed my pains? When she finished speaking, my body was taken with a force stronger than anything I'd known. Suddenly, my stomach moved; like a sea wave it rose and fell, and I shouted to the midwife, "Look, he's moving, he's coming, he's . . ."

She didn't let me finish but helped me into a squatting position on the bed. There, between the legs I thought forever closed, the baby was born. A moon head appeared, two shoulders and a tiny leaf-like hand, and the child slid out into the spread hands of the midwife.

"A girl," I whispered. "It's a girl." I could hardly believe the crumpled face belonged to my child.

The midwife clucked and said, "I've never seen such a large girl—that's what kept her so long," and she touched the baby's long body and sturdy legs.

My nurse stood by the edge of the bed and took the baby gently in her arms. The midwife cut and bound the cord, while onto the other end she tied a weight. That would help the afterbirth come out, as the midwife was not allowed to pull on the cord herself.

"Careful!" I said to my nurse. "You'll wash the child before her time." For Hsin Nai-nai was crying happily as she patted the baby dry.

Wrapping her in old, warmed clothes, my nurse spoke. "They'll say, *'Hsiao hsi'* to you, Ling; 'It's only a small happiness, this girl.' Don't listen to them. A girl is better than no child at all, and where one child grows, another will, too."

I lay back and let my head rest on the pillows, the special ones I had embroidered with longevity symbols for my bridal bed so long ago. For a moment I was sad—sad that this child, this almond-eyed beauty who came to me so late in life, should receive the sentence, "Only a small happiness."[1] A boy would have congratulations and cries of wonder and thanks; "a great happiness, a great happiness."[2] The old saying tells us that even a deformed son is better than the brightest, most skilled girl. Let them have their say; I would cherish and love this late autumn leaf, my first child. And when the time came to name her, I'd call her My Thousand Ounces of Gold to show how precious she was to me.

I had done my part and now could sleep. My nurse

---

[1] Issac Taylor Headland, *Home Life in China* (New York: The Macmillan Company, 1914), p. 10.

[2] Ibid.

would call in Li and tell my worthy husband of the birth. They could write down the hour of my child's arrival and the day, month, and year. Those eight characters of birth would be vital when it came time to match a future husband with my daughter. After the characters were recorded, my husband would send the required gift of money and a wine jar to my parents in town. That the child was a girl would be read in the paper tied around the wine jar's neck. A red paper with one end cut in slits told everyone a girl was born. Let them be busy, I thought, let them fuss and prattle—I'm going to sleep.

I slept for a day and woke to a child who no longer looked like a crumpled leaf but a real daughter. I spent all my time in bed beside her, with my nurse and Li waiting on me. My mother-in-law was not as attentive to me as before; she was disappointed in not having a grandson. My nurse told me later that Li sniffed when told the baby was a girl and said, "That's what I would expect of Ling—not the best!"

So. Let her sniff; my life was centered on the child, and I was as gay with her as children are with presents on New Year's.

Three days after the birth, we washed my child for the first time. I am not certain why we wait for the third day, but Li said we must. She holds fast to the ways of old China and fears demons as only an old woman can. I believe the waiting has something to do with avoiding evil influences.

I cannot tell all the ceremonies that followed in the days and months after my daughter's birth. I would tire of the telling, there are so many. There was the feast to celebrate the girl's first bath; magic parcels hung by my door to give her good character; and demon-catchers surrounded me and my child. Mother mine, we were not even allowed out of the birth room for the entire first month! All that is from fear of harm and evil.

But after the ceremonies—the name-giving, foretelling the child's future, praying that she be a good child, putting her under the protection of Mother—what did the future hold for my daughter?

In five years I would have to bind her feet. I remember what it is like: the toes curl under the foot; the heel is forced down; and the whole shape crushed together. I dreaded her tears and wailing, yet it must be done. All girls of good families have their feet bound. It has always been so, and only the common peasants of the fields leave them unbound, those great, splay-footed louts. When my daughter was 8, her "lillies" would be fixed in their final shape. She, too, could wear three-inch shoes, as I do, and walk like a shaking leaf.

Later, My Thousand Ounces of Gold would marry and leave our house for another's. She would belong to her husband and family and kneel before their ancestors. Like the wine jar sent from our house to announce her birth, she would be carried to a new home and put behind walls. For a woman is the *nei jen,* the inside person,[3] while men live in the outside world.

It is hard at times to live within walls, to travel outside in covered sedan chairs. We do go to festivals, to see the magnificent dragon god and the dramas of the theater. But we do not go to the cool mountains with friends to drink wine under the plum blossoms and recite poetry. We do not go to the harbor and trade with great ships from abroad. We have our children and are glad of it, as I was that day when my child bloomed from me like a magic flower on an old and withered tree.

---

[3] Ibid., p. 62.

Chapter 7
BIRTH OF THE SUN-KING

>
> Time: 1638
> Place: The castle of Saint-Germain, France
> Characters: Queen Anne, King Louis XIII, attendants, and baby

The shame of it! To have your husband brought to bed by force, carried in the arms of his good friend, the Duc de Luynes. And even to have precedence observed, with the king's *valet de chambre* going before the Duc with a lighted taper. Then to have the king deposited unceremoniously in your bed and left, like a prisoner on the block.

Queen Anne sighed, remembering that night so many years ago. She had been 18, as was her king, Louis XIII. Both had married at the age of 14, joined like two halves of a political knot and twisted together. It was no wonder the king had not consummated their marriage. After all, they were children, if not in body, certainly in mind. She, from the stern, rigid Spanish court, was protected and doll-like at the age of 14. He, from the licentious French court of the late 16th-century, revolted against it and became puritan, a little prig.

It had taken four years for their marriage to be consummated, four long years with the king's advisers, his loyal lords, his confessor, the Spanish ambassador, even the Pope's nephew begging the king to do his duty. He must produce a Catholic heir for France, secure the succession, and not insult the House of Spain by neglecting the queen.

To all their advice and entreaties, the king replied that he was young yet and must take care of his health.

The shame of it! It was not enough to have an unwilling king who must be forced to her bed. It was not enough to endure the whispers and laughter of the court. But when the marriage finally was consummated, to have messengers sent off announcing the good news! Nothing was private in the life of a king and queen; there was nothing you could call your own.

Eighteen years had passed since that night, and during that time, the king rarely came to her. It had been seven long years since the king had last slept with the queen. How could she give France the Dauphin it so desired if the king never came to her bed? Queen Anne wished she had a child for all the churches of Our Lady she had made pilgrimages to, praying to the Mother of God for a child. She had gone to every Notre Dame in France, seeking divine help for a husband who would not do his duty, for her body that was empty and barren. If she could not produce an heir, Queen Anne might be sent back in disgrace to the Spanish court, a thing she dreaded. There she would be like an extra piece of furniture, unwanted and unused.

Perhaps Our Lady heard at last the fervent prayers of Queen Anne; perhaps she rewarded the queen for twenty-two years of faithful marriage to a husband who was revolted by women, by intimate contact with them.

King Louis XIII did come to his queen again. It is said that he did so under pressure, that only the discomfort of a winter rainstorm in 1637 sent him to his queen's apartments in the Louvre. As he had no place to dine and sleep, he was forced to eat with Queen Anne and to share her bed. From that night, from the luck of a December rain and an unwell king who feared fever and rheumatism, Louis XIV was conceived.

In the weeks that followed the king's visit, the queen must have prayed and hoped for the miracle—a child. Perhaps she believed, as did many 17th-century people, that both men and women contributed seed at the moment of conception. The man's sperm was the active, reaching one; the woman's, the passive, receptive seed. However she thought of it, her prayers were answered. By late winter of 1638, she knew she was with child, and the joyous news was sent throughout France and the neighboring countries. "The queen is with child! A Dauphin is promised. Long live the queen!"

Amid the rejoicing and excitement, Queen Anne felt a great sense of relief. Now her position was secure in the French court; she could not be sent back to Spain, a disgraced, barren woman. And a queen who was carrying the heir to the throne could not be suspected of disloyalty. No longer could people whisper rumors about her, terrible rumors that she was a traitor in league with her brother, the king of Spain.

The queen was a sacred vessel bearing the future ruler of France, and she must be protected and carefully nourished. Her ladies of honor and attendants were quick to answer her every request. In a hushed atmosphere of expectation, an entire court watched the queen swell with child. The finest doctors were engaged to oversee the queen's pregnancy. In long black robes, wearing pompous, satisfied expressions, the doctors discussed the slightest symptoms of Queen Anne.

Was her color good? Did her breath come too heavily? Was her mood the result of this or that humor? Was the child's head upright in the womb or not? Everything was touched upon in the learned and grand manner of the day, and Queen Anne was lucky in her ignorance. She felt reassured by the black-robed magicians and could not know they were still unsure of many of the physical realities of pregnancy and childbirth. They could declaim in Latin; they rode fine horses and ate delicately. What more could a woman desire?

According to the custom of the 17th-century that proclaimed bleeding a remedy for everything, the queen was probably bled at regular intervals during her pregnancy; once at four and a half months, once at seven months, and again at nine months. People believed the bad blood (or old, stagnated blood) must be drawn from a person so that new, "fresh" blood could form. Did she feel weak after being bled? Probably, but like many who survived the doctors of her time, she was a hardy woman and soon recovered.

On April 22, 1638, the queen sensed the first movement of the child inside her womb. Her ladies of honor rushed to tell the doctors, they rushed to tell the king and lords, and the whole court gathered to celebrate. Fireworks were set off over the castle, and people rejoiced over the "quickened" child within the queen. Their Dauphin was alive and already asserting his kingly arms and legs.

As an added precaution during the pregnancy, the queen sent to the Capuchin monks for the girdle of the Blessed Virgin. Mary, herself, was thought to have worn this article, and it was held in reverence and awe by the people. Surely, the life-giving power of the Mother of God would be transferred to her girdle. If Queen Anne wore it, some of that power would become hers, too. Throughout her pregnancy, the queen kept the Blessed Girdle fastened around her, relying on its protection.

A little after midnight on September 5, 1638, Queen Anne felt her first labor pains. The queen's attendants hurried to her side, and the king was notified of the impending event.

Queen Anne was led to the special lying-in couch that had been set up in her warm, comfortable chambers. The couch was narrower than her ample, royal bed and was lower to the ground. It was made that way so the midwives and doctors could better attend the queen with her precious burden.

It is not known exactly what happened during the queen's hours of labor from midnight to the morning of September 5th. Most likely, her hands were held by her ladies of honor, her brow wiped with scented handkerchiefs, and her spirits refreshed with sips of red wine. Perhaps she ate a candy or two, or a bit of red meat to strengthen her.

Certainly, the queen was never left alone, not even for a

second. The birth had to be witnessed by the right people, who would make sure the queen actually bore the royal baby and did not substitute another's child in its place. For that purpose, women of the royal family and princes of the blood were called to the queen's chamber as soon as she went into labor. They probably sat on stools or chairs around the lying-in couch, near enough to witness the birth of the prince or princess.

However, the royal observers were just part of the crowd that surrounded the queen. Her ladies of honor were nearby; several doctors and assisting midwives hovered over the couch; in the antechamber were three bishops who said Mass throughout the night; and many lords of the court waited just outside the room. The royal *accoucheur* (doctor of childbirth) directed the proceedings, looking dignified in his curled wig, elegant robe, and buckled shoes. An official bag full of 17th-century remedies lay on the table beside the queen. Inside was sneezing powder to help the queen give birth, and vials of almond oil to anoint the hands of the doctor and head midwife. Boxes of powdered cumin and myrrh rested on the table, ready to dust the infant's navel cord. For the same purpose, ashes, crushed calves' feet, and powdered snail shells were at hand.

The head midwife, Dame Péronne, may have been the most knowledgeable person there. She had learned much from her years of delivering well-to-do ladies, and in the past, not so well-to-do ladies. To qualify as a midwife, Dame Péronne had to be examined by two experienced midwives, two surgeons, and one physician. That had happened long ago, and her experience was the best qualification she brought to the queen's bedside.

There is no record of what Dame Péronne actually did to assist Queen Anne during this long-awaited, miraculous event. She may have gently stroked the queen's abdomen to help in the birth; other 17th-century midwives did so. Perhaps she instructed the queen to hold her breath during the most severe pains; that was a known remedy of the time. The midwife could have raised the queen's lower body with pillows, so the child would fall easily into her hands. Perhaps the queen was put in a half-sitting position, with a bolster behind her back.

At 11:20 in the morning, Queen Anne gave birth to her child. First, a wet crown of hair appeared, a face slid out, a right shoulder, a left, and the Dauphin was born! Dame Péronne was busy receiving the baby and helping the queen; she could not fall on her knees with tears in her eyes and cry with the others, "It's a boy, a Dauphin, God be praised!"

The midwife took her precious bundle and wrapped him in a soft blanket. Wiping the mucus from his mouth and nose, Dame Péronne made certain he was alive and breathing. Nothing could go wrong with this child, and her hands trembled as she tied the umbilical cord, then cut the piece beyond the knot.

Queen Anne could hardly speak for the excitement of bearing a son, and she inwardly praised God that her child was not a girl. For she would have failed to produce the desired heir and would have to start over again on a long pregnancy.

Beyond the chamber, the door opened and the lords of the anteroom and the bishops filed in to see their new Dauphin. Even the king, adverse as he was to such earthy matters, was persuaded to come into the room, where he gazed uncertainly at his queen. Prompted by a friend, he did kiss her and thanked Queen Anne for presenting him with the needed, greatly desired heir.

As the room quickened with noise and filled with more people, the midwife and her assistant took the newborn over to the fire. There they washed the Dauphin in oil of red roses and red wine, the usual bath for wellborn infants. It would strengthen him and make him healthy. As soon as he was dry, the midwives swaddled him tightly from his toes up to his armpits in a long linen band. That would keep his body firm and upright, so he would grow into a strong man. A lace cap was placed on the prince, as no newborn could have a bare head.

Still gasping at his abrupt entrance into life, the tiny dauphin was handed to his governess and carried off to the chapel. He was surrounded by witnesses to the birth and two rows of guards. As he left the room, Queen Anne sank back into an exhausted sleep, her duty done. Although she would always have respect and honor as the mother of the Dauphin, she would be somewhat forgotten in the days to come. All attention would focus on her child, who was now being taken to his baptism.

At the chapel, one of the king's assistants dropped holy water on the newborn's forehead and pronounced him a Christian. This was done right after birth, in case the infant should die. An unbaptized soul went to purgatory, where it lingered with the almost-good pagans in a murky light. Only a baptized soul went straight to heaven. The infant was named Louis, but he would not be formally christened Louis XIV until he was 4 years old.

Outside the castle, France rejoiced at the birth of their Dauphin. They called him Louis the Godgiven, or Louis Dieudonné. He had been the result of many, many prayers, not just the queen's, but an entire nation's. He was a miracle, a gift from God sent to save France with a secure succession to the throne. In celebration of his birth, fireworks were set off throughout France. Cannons boomed from the royal castle; and in Paris, barrels of wine were set up in the streets and free wine given to all. There was dancing, singing, feasting, and Te Deums chanted in all of France. Priests offered Masses of Thanksgiving, while poets and orators wrote odes and speeches celebrating the great event. The astrologers, who were definitely believed in by 17th-century people, predicted a glorious reign for the prince. In a paroxysm of praise, one astrologer said the sun came low to the earth that day to witness the glorious birth.

And what of the new bundle of arms, legs, and pink flesh that excited such rejoicing, such outpourings of sentiment? Lying in a richly furnished chamber, Louis began his life as prince of the realm surrounded by attendants and caretakers. Every need of his was seen to: there was a cook, a laundress, two handymen, two pages, seven women to guard the sleeping infant, musicians to play him asleep, a special cradle-rocker, his own doctor, two assistant nurses, a governess, and a wet nurse.

Queens did not breast-feed their royal infants, and a woman had already been engaged to nurse Louis. She was the Dame de la Giraudière, wife to the king's attorney. But her nobility could not keep up with the Dauphin's hunger, and after three months, her milk dried up. She was put aside and another wet nurse hired.

Before a woman could be appointed *nourrice du corps* (literally, "nurse of the body"), she had to pass a strict examination. Her breasts must be firm and full of milk of the right consistency and color. It was best if she had borne her own child two months before the time she was engaged. Her complexion must be clear and her breath sweet. Although her morals and language must be approved, the woman did not have to be noble. In fact, the peasant wet nurses seemed to fare better than the first, wellborn one. A good disposition was also required in a *nourrice du corps,* as people believed her emotions could pass through her milk to the baby and might upset him.

During the days and weeks after his birth, the Dauphin was displayed to the public like an exquisite gem. Swaddled tightly from his feet up to his armpits, dressed in a fine shirt and lacy cap, Louis rested on a pillow on his governess's lap. A gilt railing separated the royal party from the rest of the room. On the other side, nobles, priests, ambassadors, statesmen, soldiers, merchants, jugglers, and the occasional peasant could come and gaze at their prince. Did he not belong to them all? In those early days, the infant Louis became accustomed to living in a crowd of people. It was good that he did so, as he would never be alone. When his swaddling clothes were changed, which was several times a day, nobles and ladies witnessed the unwrapping of the royal infant. One of the highest born handed the clean swaddling band to the dresser and felt honored by such a privilege. Another noble person held out the embroidered shirt and blessed it at the same time.

For a brief moment, the child's body was free and naked. Then the band of linen and ritual was tightened around him again. He would never know that he was a prisoner of the public and of court custom. He would never know what it was like to run free in a garden, to wear clothes that did not hamper his limbs. In time, Louis would exchange his swaddling bands for the heavy, embroidered skirts worn by noble French boys. When he was seven, he would leave the only affection he ever knew for the world of men, the training of kings. There, he would become the great Sun-King who built Versailles, patronized the arts, organized the government, built up the army and navy, and brought glory to France. Yet the Sun-King never forgot his early years in the nursery, the women who loved him as a little boy, and that time when the world of kingship was far away.

Multiple Births

Chapter 8
STRANGE BIRTH

Time: 1880
Place: Vancouver Island, British Columbia
Characters: A Nootka Indian family

Yula was worried. She had never given birth, yet she knew most women carried their first baby high and tight inside their bodies. Her body was enormous. When she stood up, her feet disappeared and Yula felt she'd been carrying a full-grown baby for months.

The Indian woman tried to reassure herself; had she not followed all rules for a woman with child? She always drank first from the water bucket, and she never ate leftovers. Eating and drinking things left sitting in their containers makes a child stay long in the womb. She avoided weaving baskets and mats, afraid that would tangle the baby's navel cord. And she never stood in a doorway, knowing her child would then linger inside. But at night, in the long house as she lay by the fire, Yula worried. What if she bore twins? What if two came forth where only one should be?

Some women desired twins and even bathed ritually in the cold lake so two would come. They considered it an honor to be the mother of twins, those special beings. Or, their husbands might want to be shamans; being the father of twins and going through the long ordeal taught a man how to call the fish upstream, how to seek visions. Yula thought such people were *wikhtin* (mad). If you bore twins, you must leave your family and village for four years. The rules governing such births were strict, and the parents could not escape them. It was as if they had met and talked with spirits, and they must be put away from ordinary people.

Yula's mother and kinswomen had already prepared the birth hut in the woods outside the settlement. All bearing had to take place away from the long houses, for fear twins or a deformed child might be born. They must not be allowed within the community, as a strange birth was dangerous to all.

When Yula's time came, she was digging clams by the lake shore with her sisters. She gasped at the quick pain and bent over, holding her hands to her body.

"Yula, Yula, it's come, it is time," her sisters cried. Like a flock of birds, they swept her up the beach, through the trees to the birth hut, all the time patting her shoulders and wondering what the child would be.

Inside the low shelter made of branches and mats, her sisters helped Yula sit on the board cushioned with shredded bark. She leaned back against the strong pole and sighed heavily; it was here at last. Soon she would know if her fears were true.

Through the long night, the Indian woman stayed by herself. Later her kinswomen and neighbors would gather outside to hear if the baby was a boy or girl. In the dark, only her mother attended her, standing beyond the door. She would not come in until her daughter was ready to give birth. Alone inside the bark shelter, holding onto the seat, Yula sighed with the wind as it blew and shuddered over the roof.

In the morning, when the light was green in the thick forest, Yula felt the child pushing downward within her body. She called out, "Mother, come to me, hurry!" and the older woman ran inside to help. As she grabbed the edge of the seat, Yula felt the head of the child straining her body to the limits. A deep breath, her mother urged her to push, and a boy fell into her mother's hands. In a short while she delivered the placenta, which was put outside the hut. As her mother tended the baby, Yula cried, "There's another inside!" She tensed her body again. A second head appeared, with two lines for eyes, a smudge for a nose, and two tiny shoulders. "It's a girl!" gasped her mother, as she took hold of the baby. In spite of her surprise, the older woman swiftly wiped the baby dry and cleaned out its mouth with her finger. Then she cut the navel cord with a mussel and wrapped the girl in soft bark.

At first, Yula's mother was dismayed. To have her daughter thrust into the forest, away from the village for four years! But ... the older woman smiled. To be the grandmother of twins was special, almost sacred. Such good fortune did not come often, and she had been a young girl the last time twins were born.

Yula was so exhausted she could hardly grieve over the twin birth. She felt torn and bruised and wanted to be put back together, as if part of her had been lost forever with the two red babies that cried and squalled nearby. If only she could begin over again, Yula thought. A short time ago she was a woman without children. Now she was the mother of twins, a creature apart, a woman with no ordinary life before her.

Outside, the usual joking and laughter were absent. The neighbors and relatives had returned to the village to tell news of the twins, to whisper it in each ear as if speaking of a spirit passing. For the Nootka believed twins came from the other world. They were relatives of the Salmon Spirits who lived under the sea and put on the bodies of fish to swim upriver and be caught by the Indians.

That was why Yula could not let the twins face each other when it came time to nurse. Always she must suckle them at the same time, with the backs of their heads touching. Otherwise, they might talk together and plan how to return to their house under the sea.

"My mother, what have I done to have this happen to me!" Yula wailed to the older woman. Later she would be brave and accepting; now she thought only of the four long, terrible years alone in the forest with her husband.

"Hush, Yula, hush." Her mother stroked her brow in the same way she soothed her grandchildren. "You must not think of the four years. Fix your mind on what you can do for the tribe. Your husband will learn to call the dog salmon and herring into our river, inside our traps and nets. Even you, my daughter, will have power—if you seek it," she added. "Have you not borne twins, have you not been touched by the spirits? Hush, then, hush."

Yula was calmed by her mother. It was true; the parents of twins were important people, a man and woman of influence. That was one reason why they must leave the village for such a long time, to learn control of that power for the good of all. And the twins must be specially cared for, separate from the village. They were dangerous, too close to the spirit world to be near ordinary people at first.

Four days after the birth, Yula and her husband went quietly, without looking back. There was only one thing she was glad of: she had no other child to leave behind. If she had children already, they would have to stay in the village for a year before rejoining their parents in the far home. Deeper and deeper into the woods went the parents with their sacred burden. Moving quietly and secretly, they came at last to the head of an inlet far from people.

That was their home for four years. By the cold green waters of the lake, Yula and her husband built a bark hut. They gathered mussels and clams, ate berries, roots, and the dried salmon their relatives brought. Each time they came, the visitors had to dress in special capes, paint their faces, and put bird down in their hair. That is how one dressed to meet a twin parent. A man or woman had to go carefully with such a one, just as a person walked carefully when near spirits.

The father of the twins took long walks in the woods, climbing steep ridges in search of visions. He was on the path of power and must learn to meet with supernatural beings and tame them.

Each night when together, Yula and her husband sang to bring the salmon and herring upriver to their people. They had the authority to call such fish. Had they not borne many, just as the fish spawned many after mating?

Twin parents could sing the fish upstream because they were as relatives of the fish, sharing in a multiple birth.

The twin boy and girl grew in a world without others. Only their parents and an occasional relative were allowed to see them, and life was a mixture of the search for food and the search for spirits.

When the family returned at last to the village, summoned by their kin, Yula and her husband were thinner and their faces had a sharp edge to them, like the crescent moon. Their long trial had brought them closer to the spirit world, and they had learned that the search for visions has its own reward.

Four years is a long time for bitter thoughts, and Yula had left hers behind long ago. She was proud of her husband, of the visions he had caught and tamed, and she had her twins—brother and sister to the Salmon Spirits. Even she, Yula, once a woman of no account, could shake her wooden rattle and summon the fish. Yula was reconciled to her life, a life that now held a new child to care for. A little girl had been born in the last year of their isolation. She was named The Salmon's Tail, as she came after the two Salmon Spirits.

And what of the twins? They grew to be shamans, a man and woman of power in the Nootka village. They could heal sickness and bring rain to their people by bathing ritually in the lake. Always they were regarded with a mixture of awe and respect. The twins were never entirely at ease in the close, intimate village of the Nootka. They had not been born into the comfortable long houses filled with the noisy chatter of many families. Instead, they were at home in the deep woods where the *ya' ai* [1] walked and the supernatural wolves vanished and reappeared. Theirs was the world of spirit voices and cries from the unseen, a world of visions and healing—only shamans and twins could walk there.

[1] The *ya' ai* were spirits who looked like hairy men with strange feathered ears.

Chapter 9
THE FEARFUL ONES

> Time: 1915
> Place: What was Tanganyika, Africa
> Characters: A Nyakyusa family and village

Lukosa stroked her belly with the satisfied gesture of a woman who has completed her purpose. Women were made to bear children; they were the "bag" which men filled with their "blood" or semen.[1] A child had sprouted in her, just as the millet and beans flourished in the dry African soil. It was the dead ancestors below the earth—the shades—who made the seed grow in the ground, who made the man's seed take root inside a woman. And as death was feared by the Nyakyusa, so birth was feared. They were but different sides of the same face.

But these thoughts were not in Lukosa, though they formed a background to her fears and desires. Her mind was on the coming birth and how she had prepared for it. She always avoided the grain fields when people were planting millet and beans. Because the seed within a woman fought seeds outside, a pregnant woman could harm grain crops.[2] Lukosa never walked by the forge of the ironsmith, as the fire within a pregnant woman fought the fire of the smith. She did not stand in her house doorway;

[1] Monica Wilson, *Rituals of Kinship Among the Nyakyusa* (London: Oxford University Press, 1952), p. 229.
[2] Ibid., page 139.

that would make the child stay in her body. And never, never did Lukosa sit too near her husband or another person. Pairing together that way gave a woman twins, and all the Nyakyusa feared the terrible fate of bearing two, like an animal.

On a warm night, when the wind rustled the leaves of the banana trees, Lukosa's pains started. This was her second birth, and she was not as afraid as she had been during her first labor. Lukosa knew what to do. She left the thatched house, certain her little boy would be safe with her co-wives, and went across the dry earth to her mother's house.

Roused from sleep, Kukwe was excited and hurried outside to ready the birth place. No woman bore children inside a house; birth was dangerous to men, and blood could harm a hunter's skill.

In back of the house, Kukwe made a soft pile of banana leaves for her daughter. There, Lukosa sat down with a groan and steadied herself for the time ahead.

Like the rain that came in gray sheets over the lake, Lukosa's pains swept over her and then retreated. In the clear spaces between, she was glad of the two women by her side—her mother and aunt. To be alone was a terrible thing, and their company and low talk made the hours pass more easily.

At dawn, Lukosa gave birth to a baby girl, and in a short time delivered another girl. They were identical twins and so shared the same placenta.

Her mother and aunt were too busy to talk at first, as they wiped the infants, cut their cords, and tied them with different kinds of bark to show who was first- and who second-born. When Kukwe finished with the babies, she looked at her daughter and exclaimed, "Two," in a low, fearful voice. "Daughter, daughter, how could there be two? Did you not . . . ?" But Kukwe stopped in midsentence. It was not Lukosa's fault she had borne twins. It was the ancestor Kyala and the dead below who made twins grow inside a woman.

What should have been a time of rejoicing became a

time of mourning. It was as if someone had died, and all the fear and pollution of a too-close contact with the shades was on them now. If Kyala and the shades were present in one birth, how much more so were they in a double birth.

"*Ilipasa* [unnatural birth], *ilipasa,*" moaned Lukosa. But there was no time to comfort her. Everyone could moan over the twin birth that was like a disease. All their relatives would have to be purged of its infection, and much had to be done.

Two huts must be built: one for Lukosa and one for Bapala, the unfortunate father of the twins. His brothers worked swiftly to erect the shelters before night came, as the mother and her two infants could not be seen by the village. This held true for the father, too, though his seclusion was not as strict as the mother's.

By nightfall the huts were ready, and Lukosa moved slowly into her special shelter. On the earth floor was a pile of leaves for a bed and a fire to warm her through the night. Her mother had thoughtfully put down a pot of hot food. Lukosa could not cook for herself or her husband during the next month; instead, her relatives would bring them food. They could do nothing in the weeks ahead but sit and wait for the time of infection to pass. During this terrible month, it was as if they were surrounded by the shades, as if the dead clung to them like an evil fog. Just as mourners stayed unwashed after a death, so Lukosa and her husband could not wash themselves. Neither she nor Bapala could call out if they wanted anything, but must talk in soft whispers. Twins were fragile babies with a loose hold on this world, and the loud voices of the father or mother might frighten them away or harm them. Also, the Nyakyusa felt parents of twins were like the animals that gave birth to litters. Since animals could not talk, the parents of twins were kept from normal speech.

Two weeks passed, bringing hot, dry weather and taking away one of the twin girls. Like a sigh in the night she left, a tiny breath of a person who could not suck enough strength from her mother's breast.

Lukosa was relieved when the frail one died. It was often

so with twins, and she had not hoped both would survive. Now she only had one to care for, but that did not change the rules governing her isolation. Even if one child died, twin parents were still dangerous. They were people of power, with a fierce blood in them to have borne two. Such terrible fertility (produced by the dead) could make a relative's legs and stomach swell, could make their bowels run. These diseases were only prevented by putting "the fearful ones" away from the village, and later, by purifying all villagers with special medicines.

A month after the abnormal birth, a tall, striking woman with brass rings around her waist came to Lukosa. She was the doctor who would cleanse the twin parents and help keep their infection from spreading to relatives and the village cattle.

Outside the isolation huts, the doctor built a fire and stirred her medicine in an iron pot. The kin of the twin parents gathered and stood talking nearby. The doctor took up a frayed bamboo shoot and dipped it in the pot, calling, "Come, it is ready," urging the reluctant ones to be purified. One by one, the woman splashed the scalding liquid on the relatives' legs. All were burned by it—women, small children, babies, and men. They screamed and jumped at the pain, but it must be done, had to be endured. How else could the danger from the abnormal birth be taken away? Just as that event had "burned" the relatives with power and danger, so the doctor burned them to drive away infection.[3]

Two weeks later, Bapala's brother set fire to the old isolation huts and a new one was built. Lukosa, Bapala, and their little girl sat inside, allowed at last to be together. They had been washed for the first time in a month, their heads shaved of hair, and their bodies rubbed with medicine. The horror of that strange birth was almost gone from them; it had been burned in the fire, washed, and shaved away. The parents were no longer dangerous to each other and could sit and whisper together in the hut.

As a ritual sign they could be near each other again,

---

[3] Ibid., p. 171

Lukosa and her husband made love on a special bed prepared by the doctor. Their making love did more than banish the long month of isolation; it helped to drive away the dead. It was as if the husband said to the shades, "You were with me and my wife during that month in the hut; now she's mine again. Go back to your home in the earth, leave us."

Outside the hut, the kin gathered again to be purified by the doctor. All of the women had washed and shaved themselves, paring away the "dirt" of the abnormal birth from their bodies. The doctor went from one person to another, putting medicine on their foreheads. That allowed them to talk and meet with the twin parents; it protected the relatives from their power. Then Bapala came out of the hut and took up a bamboo shoot. He dipped it into the hot medicine and splashed it over his relatives' legs, just as the doctor had done two weeks before. That special liquid would keep their legs from swelling and their bowels from running. At last the people were truly clean and free of the dreaded shades.

Lukosa jumped to her feet and ran out of the hut with her baby girl. Bapala grabbed his spear and shield and danced a warrior dance, the dance of a man who puts the dead back where they belong, who fights their terrible power with loud cries and a sharp spear. Together, all the relatives ran through the village shouting, "We are clean, we are clean!"

The dangerous period was over, and they could feast on meat and plantains, drinking specially brewed beer with medicine in it. Only two things remained to be done. First, Lukosa and Bapala must leave a food offering in the groves of their ancestors. Then, in the near future, Bapala must see to the herds of the village. He would sprinkle all the cattle with medicine to make certain they would not bear twins or suffer from purging. Even animals could be affected by the power of a twin birth, and they must be protected.

The isolation and ordeal of the twin parents were over. They could return to their normal lives with only a few restrictions. But always they would be looked upon as "others": people who had borne many, like animals, and people who had been so close to the shades that they had borne two instead of one.

These are just two ways in which a culture may deal with twins. Both the Nootka Indians and the African Nyakyusa treat the birth of twins as an abnormal, dangerous event. In one, the danger of the event is transformed into a power to be used. Here, the Nootka parents learn to control the fish supply, while the twins become shamans who can control the weather. With the Nyakyusa, there is no idea that the power of a twin birth can be channeled. It is seen as a disease, a contagion, a horror to be put out of sight and then washed away.

This way of seeing twins has an extreme end—killing one or both of the babies immediately after birth. Among most hunting cultures, where tribes are on the move and food and game are scarce, two infants are a terrible burden on their mother. To avoid such a hardship, one or both babies may be strangled, suffocated, or simply left to die. Tribes don't make the conscious statement, "Twins are one too many for the mother and must be killed." Instead, magical or religious reasons are given for the infanticide: twins are evil or abnormal; they come from the unseen spirit world; they are like a disease or an illness; human beings don't give birth to two, only animals do. Among the tribes in which twin infants were not allowed to live were the Arunta (Aborigines) of Australia, the Mbouti Pygmies of Africa, and some Eskimo groups.

But not all cultures fear or detest twins; some welcome them and pray for their lucky birth. The Yoruba of West Africa feel twins are very special, almost divine. It is good the Yoruba value twins highly, for their rate of twinning is the highest in the world, almost one out of every twenty-five births.[4] These twins have their own god who watches

---

[4] Amram Scheinfeld, *Twins and Supertwins* (New York: J.B. Lippincott Company, 1967), p. 62.

over them and guards their health. Whenever a twin dies, a wooden carving is made and given to the surviving child. He or she carries the figure about, dressing, "feeding," even washing it. The carving is meant to comfort the remaining twin, and also to be a resting place for the dead one's spirit.

Among the Lele of Southwest Africa, twins are said to be gifts from the spirits. The parents automatically become Twin Diviners, members of a special cult called Twin Parents. They have power to foretell the future and to bring good hunting and crops to the village. Because they have been so fertile in bearing two, the parents can influence the fertility of the entire village.

Africans are not the only people to make twin parents members of a distinct group. In America, mothers can belong to an organization called the Mothers of Twins club. There, women give support and advice on the difficulties of caring for two. But it is the birth of triplets, quadruplets, and more that are treated as news items in American newspapers. Pictures are taken of the tiny matching infants, with the father looking on (worrying about the bills), and the mother beaming. They are feted, and collections of money are taken to help with the babies' care. All in all, a minor miracle has taken place, and the parents are honored and also teased. The jokes tease the father about his immense potency and the mother about her marvelous powers. Even we still wonder at the fertility of a multiple birth.

Most cultures mark multiple births in special ways. Often, the rites performed for twins include any abnormal birth, such as children born fanny-first (breech birth), infants with cauls, or children born with the navel cords around their necks. The basic feeling about such events is that they are unnatural. And the parents are seen to be especially powerful and/or dangerous people.

Many hunting and non-urban cultures feel that to bear two, even three, makes you like an animal with a litter. Some groups react with disgust, while others welcome the unique fertility of twin parents. So the Nootka linked twin parents to their fish supply and made sure the couple did their best to keep the salmon and herring running upstream.

Again and again the question arises: "How can two be born? We're made to bear one." The mystery of a twin birth can lead to some interesting explanations of how two are produced. One African tribe, the Kaffirs, punished the mother of twins as an adulteress. Twins were thought to have two fathers, and the mother was to blame.

Some people feel the gods or spirits create twins, that growing two inside is like a supernatural conception. The Nuer of Africa call twins Children of God, and they are linked to the sky. Often twins are believed to have power over the weather, especially rain and storms. Such influence comes from their being produced by a sky spirit.

Other cultures may struggle with the question: "Are twins one person or two?" It is easy to see why people ask that question with identical twins. For the African Nuer, twins had one social personality. They must be treated the same and married on the same day. If one twin died, he or she was not mourned. As long as one survived, the whole person was considered to be alive.

Many societies treat twins exactly alike, as if the twins are truly one. The Dahomey of Africa dress twins alike, and the same gift must be given to each. Americans often treat identical twins as one person, dressing them in matching outfits, calling them by similar names, even punishing them simultaneously when young.

If people have a hard time deciding if twins are one or two, apparently animals do also. Dogs cannot tell identical twins apart at first, and are confused by their scent.

When twins happen to be male and female, a culture may consider them to be "married." One Bantu tribe called them "newly-weds," and the ancient Japanese married the boy and girl twins when they were grown.

If twins are believed to be two separate people, they may be seen as enemies and rivals. In the Book of Genesis, Jacob and Esau fought in their mother's womb and were born enemies. One was a smooth man, Jacob, and the other a hairy man; one a hunter, and one a tent-dweller. They established separate nations. In Greek mythology, the twins Romulus and Remus founded Rome and fought as they marked the boundaries of the city. Remus was killed during the bitter struggle. In other myths, twins may follow completely different, opposing paths. One is mortal, while the other is immortal. One plays the lyre, and the other carries stones. One heals blindness, and the other inflicts it.

It seems that twins are either regarded as one person (if the same sex), married (if opposite sexes), or as hostile rivals. Very few cultures see twins as two separate people with individual interests, who can still be friends.

Whether twins are considered dangerous or helpful, the same person or two, created by the gods above or the shades below, like animals or not, most cultures of the past agreed that twins were unusual, often powerful beings. The parents who bore such oddities had to be treated in special ways, for they were either fearfully or joyfully fertile. And the twins themselves? They may have been despised, put outside the community, even killed, or welcomed with dances and gay celebrations as Children of God, the special ones, the magic two.

Birth in Modern Times

Chapter 10
BIRTH IN AMERICA

Time: 1977
Place: Massachusetts, U.S.A.[1]
Characters: A man and wife

"Guess what, mom? I'm pregnant!" The voice coming over the phone was happy and excited.

The reply was immediate. "That's wonderful, Joanne, just wonderful! And about time, too, I might add," the woman chuckled.

Joanne did not respond. She was 30 years old and she knew her long years of childlessness had worried her mother. The question had started when Joanne was 24, two years married. "When are you going to have a family, Joanne? I'd so love to have a grandchild, and now's just the time for you."

What did they know? Joanne thought. "I'll choose the right time for me," she'd answered fiercely, clinging to her power of choice. For she could choose; that was the big difference between Joanne and her mother and grandmother.

Joanne's mother had had three children in rapid succession during the 1940's. She had given birth to her first child nine months after the wedding, delivering under heavy

---

[1] This is about one experience in one American hospital; it is not meant to be representative of every American woman's labor and delivery. Some women have far better experiences in hospitals; others have far worse.

sedation—the favored "twilight sleep" of the day. Wives were expected to have babies and did; if they had doubts, they were rarely expressed.

And her grandmother? Joanne remembered the thin, dry woman who had borne eight children, four at home, four in the hospital. Contraceptives had not been widely available in her day, and a woman had no real power over her body—when to have children, when not to. Her grandmother could not remember the details of the eight births. When she spoke of her pregnancies, it was as if she were another person, a far-away ghost unconnected to that young woman with a swollen belly.

Joanne brought her mind back to her own mother talking cheerfully on the other end of the phone.

"Remember not to eat any fatty foods, dear, and not to go skiing or horseback riding. And I'll come and help after the baby's born. Don't forget to call Dr. Wilmont; he's the best obstetrician in town."

"Yes, mom, I already have a doctor, mom," Joanne answered and ended the conversation with a promise to call next week and tell how she "felt."

"This is going to be a long seven months," Joanne said to her husband that night at dinner. (She had gone for a pregnancy test only after two months of missed periods.)

"How so?" said Steve. He was still in a state of shocked excitement about Joanne's pregnancy and had trouble speaking whole sentences. Would he be a good father? his mind raced. Could he support a child? What about medical bills; it now cost about $1,500 to have a child.

Joanne continued. "Well, I feel I have to fight for control over this baby. My mother tells me what to eat, what to do, and my doctor already speaks of this baby as if it's his. Whose baby is this, anyway?" And Joanne burst into tears.

"There, there," Steve patted her awkwardly across the dinner table. "It's just hormones, dear. All women get upset during pregnancy."

"But I'm not all women, Steve, I'm me!" and she jumped up from the table and ran outside. Here, under the black March sky, she could own her body again. She spread her fingers over her stomach; nothing to feel yet from the outside. Only, in the morning, there was a heaviness inside and her breasts hurt.

She had friends who had hated pregnancy, who disliked the thought of their bodies being "taken over." "It felt like a tumor," said one. Another thought of the fetus as "a parasite feeding on me."

Joanne did not share those feelings, but she was fiercely protective of the small life within. From reading books about pregnancy and birth, Joanne knew the child at eight weeks was the length of her thumbnail (one inch) and looked like a tiny doll with an enormous head. She followed the progression of photographs religiously as the weeks passed, trying to imagine the embryo as it became more and more human. It had minute ears, eyes shut tight at first, a bald head, and arms and legs that kicked within the warm fluid of the amniotic sac. Inside, as it grew, the baby would suck its thumb, scratch its belly, and turn somersaults.

The third month of her pregnancy went by with only a little morning sickness, and Joanne entered the second trimester (the fourth through sixth months). She visited her doctor once a month to have her weight, blood pressure, and urine checked. This was to make certain she did not gain too much weight and that she had no urinary infections. The doctor also listened to the fetus's heartbeats and felt its position inside her womb, checking that the child was developing as it should.

Joanne carefully watched everything she ate: not too much liquor; no smoking; plenty of fruits, vegetables, and protein. No drugs at all, not even an aspirin did she allow herself. Joanne remembered the babies with flipper arms who had been born after their mothers took the drug Thalidomide, and she feared to take any medicine whatsoever.

She continued her life as before, walking every morning to the school where she taught. Joanne was determined her body would be strong, ready for birth when it came. At night, naked before the mirror, she did deep kneebends, watching her belly rise and fall. It was rounder now, taut and hard as a basketball. It was the first unclothed pregnant body she'd ever seen in her life. Pregnant women wore loose tunics and dresses; and at the beach (not many swam), frilly bathing suits draped their large figures.

"How can I be thirty years old and never have seen what women really look like under those maternity dresses—those tents?" Joanne asked her husband. "It's insane! We ... we hide it away like it's a sickness or a funny crooked limb we don't want anyone to see."

"That's true," mused Steve. "Do you know, I've never seen anything being born? Not even a cat or a dog?" They laughed ruefully at each other, at their shared ignorance.

"Seventh month!" Joanne said proudly and marked its beginning on the calendar. "Pretty soon we can start classes."

"But it's not for another eight weeks," protested Steve.

"I know, but it's time to go and learn the exercises."

They had decided to have the baby through natural childbirth, using the Lamaze method of controlled breathing. Many obstetricians preferred women to use anesthesia and pain-killers during the birth, feeling they made it easier for the mother and infant. Yet many of these drugs also entered the child's body and could slow its breathing and heartrate. Balancing her own desire for a painless birth and her desire for an alert baby, Joanne chose not to use drugs.

But it was only after long and careful thought that Joanne and Steve decided to use Lamaze. In the months before her due date, they both read about different methods of giving birth, searching out the right one for them. Joanne considered childbirth through hypnosis, where you learned to make your hand numb and then transfer that numbness to your belly, erasing the pain. Since there were no doctors trained in hypnosis in their town, they abandoned that idea.

There was the Leboyer method of birth, where lights and sound were dimmed in the delivery room and the newborn was put immediately on the mother's stomach. A warm bath and a calm atmosphere eased the infant's transition into a harsh, strange world. Although the local hospital did allow some of the French doctor's methods, some were considered unsafe—it would be a compromise.

Joanne explored the idea of home birth with Steve, trying to persuade him to agree to it. She liked the thought of giving birth in her own bed, surrounded by warm and familiar faces. But Steve felt otherwise.

"I know it's your decision, Joanne, but I'd feel too worried. I just don't think it's safe with the first, with you being an older mother."

"But in England they do it all the time, and nurse-midwives deliver the babies safely. Fewer babies die *there* than they do here!"

"That's England; we don't have the medical backup for home birth that the Europeans do," Steve pointed out. "I know ninety-five percent of all births are normal," he stalled her objection, "but you might just be in that five percent, with the baby in the wrong position, or with a long and difficult labor."

"Well, maybe you're right," Joanne agreed, secretly relieved. She wasn't ready for home birth yet, she realized. Maybe with the second child, when she'd learned what to expect.

Joanne also talked with her friends about their experiences with different hospitals and doctors. One woman had given birth with the vacuum bubble, which she described as "a big bowl that fits over your abdomen and pubic area." The air was sucked out, and the decreased pressure under the bubble made it easier for the uterus to contract. Somehow, the vacuum bubble had not caught on as a general aid to laboring women, and the local hospital did not have one.

Joanne thought of the other cultures she'd read about in her search for different ways of giving birth: the New Guinea tribeswoman bearing a child inside a hut on a cold hillside; the Zuñi woman who was surrounded by family as she gave birth; the Chinese woman who struggled alone, relying on a magic puppet show to ease her pains; the

Greek woman who delivered on a birth stool, supported by midwives; and the Eskimo woman who gave birth on the floor, with the husband squeezing the child out.

And their way—the American way? Joanne knew there were good reasons for having skilled professionals attend birth, for being in clean surroundings, for medical backup when needed. Infant mortality had been greatly reduced over the years, and women were healthier after birth. But this elaborate procedure—the instruments, the sterile sheets, the drugs, the masked doctor and nurses—was part of her culture, just as the Zuñi sand bed, Chinese puppets, and bewigged French doctor were part of other cultures. Though Joanne was glad not to give birth on a cold hillside, she missed the intimacy, the closeness of the other cultures. Perhaps we've gone too far in the other direction, she thought, in our desire to make birth safe and easy.

At the end of the seventh month, Steve and Joanne went to the Lamaze class at their local hospital. There she learned how to breathe deeply and slowly for the early stage of labor; how to do fast, shallow breathing as the labor progressed; how to "pant-blow" during the hardest part of labor; and when to help push, as the baby began to leave the uterus. Together they watched a film on childbirth and, for the first time in their lives, saw a baby being born.

At nine months Joanne was ready, tired of waiting for the baby. At one time she'd been afraid of deformities. "Will he or she be normal?" she'd asked her doctor. And he had taken her hand and let her feel, "There, that's an elbow—that bump's a leg, and you can feel his head through here," pressing her fingers against a hard, round object. Although it seemed her child was a puzzle of unconnected pieces, Joanne was reassured they were all there.

At least twenty times in the past month Joanne had asked Steve, "How can you still love me?" sticking out her stomach even further. It was ridiculous, this large belly; she wasn't a woman but a cow!

But Steve had convinced her. "You're beautiful, it's beautiful, I like you big."

"There's so much they don't tell you," Joanne complained.

"Like?"

"Like the fact my belly button has popped out and is sore, like how much I sweat, like how my legs hurt!"

"You're forgetting the other part," he said, rubbing the small of her back where it ached. "About how you'd never felt so alive before; how proud you feel of growing this child; and remember what your mom said?"

"I remember," Joanne laughed. Her mother had patted Joanne's stomach and said wonderingly to her own husband, "Our genes are flowing through this child, John—our genes!"

Joanne felt connected, part of a stream of heredity that went way back into the past. And this, this round self she carried before her? It was her gift to the future, her link with times to come.

On a warm night in October, Joanne woke from an uneasy sleep. Her back ached and her belly was stretched and taut. There—there it was again. A tug, a pulling, a . . .

"It's a contraction, Steve!" she shouted in his ear.

Steve sat straight up in bed, stared wildly at her, and reached for the phone.

"No, no, not yet, Steve! It's just started."

They both lay down again, and Joanne took her luminous watch to time the contractions. Fifteen minutes apart—it would be hours yet.

Five long hours later, Joanne and Steve drove to the hospital. Now the contractions were five minutes apart, and her doctor had said she could come in. Steve signed the necessary papers at the admitting desk, while Joanne breathed deeply, inhaling and exhaling for the first stage of labor.

A nurse took her to a labor room, a small white cell with

two beds in it, and gently undressed her. Her clothes were taken away, and she was given a white hospital gown that left her back cold and naked. She climbed onto the bed, and the nurse propped her back with pillows.

"I'm glad you don't shave our pubic area and give us enemas anymore," Joanne said to the nurse.[2]

The nurse smiled and said, "So am I. I had my babies in the 'old days,' and I can tell you, it could be unpleasant. I didn't have *my* husband by me fifteen years ago!"

Through the next fourteen hours of labor the couple worked together: Joanne breathing to control the labor pains; Steve wiping her brow, timing the contractions, and encouraging her. The nurse rubbed her back, gave her ice chips to suck on, and kept Joanne comfortably supported with pillows. As Joanne's pains increased, the nurse suggested she take some Demerol. "It will help dull the pain," she said. A "relaxing shot" was also offered, but Joanne shook her head. This might be the only time she would give birth, and she would go through it as she was. When she felt pain, she would feel all of it; when she felt joy, she would let it rush through her. Nothing would dull or change those sensations. Joanne also knew that once you took a pain-killing drug, it could be harder to control the contractions with breathing. You weren't alert enough to stay on top of them.

Across the hall Joanne could hear other women in labor. Some called back and forth to each other: "Keep up your breathing!" Or, "Don't work so hard; lie back and rest between contractions." There was a sharing, a camaraderie in the maternity wing, and the nurses seemed happier to be here than in any other part of the hospital.

Her doctor arrived and came in to examine Joanne during the last two hours. "Five centimeters dilated," he said, at first, noting how far her cervix had widened. "Seven centimeters dilated," one and a half hours later. And finally, "It's time, wheel her in. You're doing well,

---

[2] Some hospitals still "prep" women for birth in this way.

Joanne," he said, praising her as if she were an athlete running a race.

Joanne had to leave her bed and climb onto another before she could be wheeled into the delivery room. Though the nurses helped her, she resented it and complained to the doctor, "How can you make me move at a time like this?"

He laughed and patted her hand; most women in the late stages of labor were "cranky," as he put it, and he was used to it.

In the delivery room, bright spotlights shone down on the bed, and masked nurses stood ready to help the doctor. Joanne changed to another bed and lay back as her feet were put up in the metal stirrups.

"I hate these things," she said between breaths, protesting the stirrups. It was part of the hospital routine she could not change, a device originally invented for doctors who did rectal operations. Lying on her back with her feet up was convenient for the doctor but not always so for the laboring mother. The weight of the mother's uterus and baby (almost eleven pounds) pressed on the body's major aorta, cutting off the blood supply to her uterus, the baby, and her legs. Gravity worked against the mother and made it harder to push the baby out.

"You're doing fine, dear," said one of the nurses and held her hand.

Joanne couldn't even see the lower half of her body. Sterile, green sheets were draped over her belly and legs—all to protect the newborn from infection. Joanne felt disconnected; her head was at one end, while this intense, powerful activity was going on at the other end.

"Now," the doctor said, "do you feel like pushing?"

Joanne didn't answer, ovewhelmed by the need to bear down, to push with her entire body.

"Good girl!" the doctor said. "Again, push, push!"

A nurse said excitedly, "There, I see some hair; it's the head!"

The doctor made a small slit in the flesh below the birth-opening to ease the baby out. Joanne looked up in the mirror above the table and saw a dark, wet head pushing against her vulva.

"Now, stop working and ease the baby out—gently, gently," the doctor said.

"Use rapid breathing," Steve urged, and Joanne panted, trying to control her desire to push as she felt herself widen and stretch, felt heat, and the head came out. Its mouth opened and a cry escaped, startled and angry. Quickly, the doctor suctioned the mucus from the baby's mouth and nose.

Then—a shoulder. The doctor slipped his finger under the armpit and helped gently. Another shoulder appeared, and a baby girl slid out into the doctor's gloved hands.

As Steve and Joanne laughed and cried together ("It's a girl! Isn't she beautiful? Look at all that hair!"), the doctor put the baby on Joanne's stomach on top of the sterile sheets.

"Don't touch her now," he warned Joanne.

She had to fight the urge to stroke her baby, to touch the soft skin. Instead, Joanne kept her hands under the sheets and watched as the doctor took the baby up, clamped and cut the umbilical cord. Then a nurse carried her over to a small crib under a heat lamp. There she was wrapped in a blanket, and her color, heartbeat, reflexes, and muscle tone were tested. If anything were wrong with the baby, this was the time to find and deal with it. Silver nitrate drops were put in the child's eyes as a protection against blindness, should the mother have syphilis.

The tiny girl was then given to Steve. Carefully, as if she were a piece of blown glass, he held her out at arm's length to show Joanne. She was not allowed to touch the baby until the placenta was delivered, her episiotomy sewed up, and her body cleaned with Phisohex, a special soap.

"So much washing!" Joanne said to herself, thinking of Lady Macbeth. She couldn't escape the feeling that she had a disease, was contaminated, and that the child—*her* baby—must be protected from her.

"Congratulations," said the doctor and kissed Joanne as

she was wheeled off to the recovery room. Steve went with her.

There the baby was brought a short time later and given to Joanne to breast-feed. The nurse cautioned Joanne, as she reached out eagerly, "Don't kiss her on the face, dear, only behind her ears."

Joanne was so glad to have her baby that she didn't protest and kissed the baby behind one crumpled ear.

After the child had nursed, she was taken away to the nursery. She would stay there for the next twelve hours until the early morning feeding.

"Do you think we'll recognize her?" Joanne worried. They'd had so little time with her, not enough to know her face.

"I think so, honey, don't worry."

In a way, Joanne was glad to be free of the baby. She wanted to sleep, to let her body knit back together again. But she missed her child. After all that work, the labor, not to have the baby by her side! Her body and her arms were empty.

"Hold me until I go to sleep," she asked her husband, and he cradled her head. Joanne was a new mother, but there was nothing she wanted so much as her own mother, to be held and comforted.

"There," Steve stroked her wet hair, "there."

*The Population Problem:
Both Sides*

Chapter 11
CONTRACEPTION THROUGH HISTORY

> "Take a square foot or more sheet of paper on which silkworm eggs have been hatched, burn to an ash and pulverize. After childbirth mix this in liquor and take. Those with impoverished blood will not again become pregnant for the rest of their lives."[1]

> Cut you the foot from one live female weasel and give it to a woman to wear round her neck. While wearing it, she will not bear children. Yet remove it, and she will conceive.

Both of these hopeful recipes for preventing conception come from widely different cultures in different times.* Yet they share a common theme that is found throughout history—the desire to control fertility. As men and women have yearned for children, praying at the foot of sacred mountains, sacrificing at the temple of Mother, so too have they wanted to block conception, to choose when they will bear children.

---

[1] Norman E. Himes, *The Medical History of Contraception* (New York: Schocken Books, 1970), p. 109.

* *None*, I emphasize none, of the ancient contraceptive methods described in this chapter should be used by *anyone*. Many are very unsafe and most are ineffective. There is *no* substitute for a doctor's supervision and professional advice and care.

The earliest attempts at contraception can only be guessed. Did prehistoric men and women say magic charms or use herbs to prevent pregnancy? We cannot know. Infant deaths were probably quite high among Neanderthal and Cro-Magnon people, and the life-span of both men and women was short (around 35 years). Perhaps they felt no need to limit the number of births. Instead, they may have spent more time in magic chants and gathering herbs to make sure they *did* have children.

However, hunting/gathering tribes known to researchers at the end of the last century and the beginning of this one did use certain contraceptive measures, despite the fact that infant mortality was often quite high in these groups. Perhaps some of the means used by these tribes were also discovered by our Cro-Magnon ancestors 30,000 years ago.

How did tribal peoples prevent conception? Most often, magical charms, songs, amulets, and herbs made up contraceptive techniques. But there were also comparatively effective ways—some of them quite ingenious. In discussing the means other cultures used to block pregnancy, it is important to remember this: how people prevent conception depends upon their knowledge of how conception occurs.

Some Central Australian tribes believed that the souls of babies rested in special stones and trees, waiting for young, desirable women to pass by. If a woman did not want more children but had to walk near those spirit centers, she might have tried fooling the babies. Bending over and hobbling past, she would say in a shaky voice, "Keep away from me; I am an ancient one."

Other magical ways to block conception included knot-tying and rites using infertile objects. Tying knots to induce sterility was a custom found throughout the world. The belief was that the knot outside a woman acted as a knot inside her, preventing pregnancy.

Because stones are lifeless, unable to reproduce themselves, they were important in magic rites to stop conception. The Maori of New Zealand thought stones could make a woman infertile, while a tribe from Eddystone

Island asked that a woman be barren "as the stone on the mountain." [2]

The dead were also part of contraceptive rites, as people believed their lifelessness could be absorbed by others. A woman of a Moroccan tribe might have stepped three times over a fresh grave to prevent pregnancy. Or she could drink the water in which a corpse had been washed.

Herbs and roots played a major role in tribal contraception, and some were believed to induce abortion. Certain American Indians had a wide knowledge of plants meant to prevent pregnancy. No thorough study has been done to determine if any of these plants actually worked for the women who used them. A few almost certainly were effective, but the majority were probably more "magical" than practical.

How was this contraceptive information spread inside different tribes? Often the people who passed on such techniques were the midwives and medicine women of the tribe. Besides attending births, they sometimes helped with abortions. Among one tribe of New Guinea, a special woman was called in to make another sterile. This contraceptive "office" was hereditary and passed down from mother to daughter. The medicine woman would burn certain herbs, rub the abdomen of the mother, and chant charms to make her barren.

Yet magical rites were only part of the methods used by hunting/gathering groups; other techniques probably did prevent pregnancy in some instances. Some tribes experimented with ways to block a woman's cervix so sperm could not enter. Women of the Kasai Basin in Central Africa inserted a cervical plug made of chopped grass. The Dahomeys of West Africa made a barrier from a crushed root. Both methods could be very harmful to women and were unsafe.

The women of Easter Island knew how to cover the uterine mouth with a bit of seaweed or algae. Yet the most ingenious device was found by the Djukas, a black tribe in

---

[2] Ibid., p. 27

South America descended from slaves. A Djuka woman sometimes put a vegetable seed pod inside her vagina to contain the semen.

Douches (liquids used to wash sperm from the vagina) were also known to certain groups. In South America, another black tribe descended from slaves mixed lemon juice with a liquid made from nut husks. Since citric acid will kill sperm, this mixture could have been effective.

Occasionally, a kind of violent massage was performed on women who wished to be sterile. In Java, a midwife might rub a woman's abdomen and then try to push the uterus backward. This was extremely painful, dangerous, and probably useless, as a tipped uterus does not prevent conception.

There are more certain ways of limiting family size. While abortion and infanticide are not contraception, they are part of people's desire to control their fertility. For some groups, they were almost the only way to limit births. Infanticide was practiced by some Aborigine tribes in times of hunger or drought. Abortion was also known and occasionally performed by the Aborigines, who used sharp instruments and, possibly, special plant drugs to end the pregnancy.

Abstinence (refraining from intercourse) was widely practiced by many tribes, and the rules of group enforced it in different cases. Among the Arapesh of New Guinea, the parents of an infant were not allowed to make love until the child walked. This kept the mother from the burden of caring for two babies at one time. Most hunting/gathering groups had rules governing parental intercourse. Parents might be forbidden to make love until the child could walk (around one year), or until the child was weaned (sometimes three years).

In tribes where taboos did not forbid intercourse after a baby's birth, prolonged nursing could prevent conception at times. If a mother breast-fed her child for two years (giving the baby little other food), she would be somewhat protected from pregnancy. Nursing can hinder ovulation, especially in the months right after birth.

Withdrawal of the male organ (or penis) from the vagina before the ejaculation of semen was also known to some groups, particularly African tribes. Yet it probably was not as widespread as it could have been. Certain tribes were unsure how conception actually took place, or felt that intercourse was only one step in creating a child, that special rites and the actions of spirits were equally important.

In recorded history, the early urban civilizations of the world discovered their own methods—some like the ones used by hunting/gathering tribes, others quite different. The earliest written sign of men's and women's desire to control childbearing is found with the Egyptians. The Petri Papyrus, written in 1850 B.C., contains prescriptions for blocking conception, and marvelous and horrible they can be!

Take you some crocodile dung, mix it with honey to a paste, and put at the mouth of the uterus, suggests one recipe. Another mentions covering the cervix with gum, probably taken from the gum acacia tree. Did these prescriptions work? Honey may have been useful, as was gum, for a sticky or gummy mixture can prevent sperm from entering the uterus. The use of dung would have been dangerous, as the bacteria it contained might have caused an infection.

The Ebers Papyrus of 1550 B.C. is the first document known to recommend a lint tampon; it was soaked in a herbal liquid and honey. The liquid was made from acacia tips which, if they are allowed to ferment, produce lactic acid—a spermicide. How did the Egyptians discover that an acacia solution could kill sperm? We don't know, but it is fascinating that some of the earliest methods of contraception are adapted and still used today. Lactic acid is one of the active ingredients in modern spermicidal jellies.

Apparently, women may have been made into "female eunuchs" in later Egyptian times to become concubines for kings. A woman's ovaries were removed to make her sterile—if she survived the surgery!

Abortion was also known to the Egyptians and written

about in the Ebers Papyrus. Some scholars think they approved of it, while others feel they condemned it.

The ancient Hebrews practiced some forms of contraception, and the Talmud (the major body of Jewish law) even specifies which women must use "a sponge." This seems to be the earliest written reference to a sponge or spongy material used to block the cervix. It probably was made of wool or a kind of cloth, and may have been covered with oil or honey to make it more effective. This form of contraception was prescribed for nursing mothers and girls who were considered too young (11–12) to bear children. Especially interesting is the recognition that pregnancy can be undesirable for or harmful to women under certain conditions; concern is shown for a woman's health. Because the Bible and the Talmud command a man to "be fruitful," all responsibility for contraception was placed on the woman.

Two other methods mentioned in early Hebraic writings were a liquid made from roots that was meant to sterilize a woman, and withdrawal. This was condemned by some Rabbis, while others recommended withdrawal to prevent conception in nursing mothers.

Greek and Roman writers combine useful information with wildly ineffective methods. Yet Greek physicians did real pioneering work in discovering successful contraception. Throughout their writings, there is a real concern with limiting family size. Both Plato and Aristotle wanted laws regulating the number of children a couple could have.

Some of the more effective kinds of ancient contraception were these: soft wool moistened with oil or honey and placed at the uterine opening; putting alum on the cervix (this stinging chemical shrinks the uterine mouth and may kill sperm); blocking the uterus with cedar-gum; making a cervical cap from beeswax; and douching with a liquid made from salt or alum.

However, the Greek and Roman approaches to contraception also included these methods: wearing an amulet of mule's earwax (since mules were infertile, a part of them was believed to confer sterility); drinking asparagus juice; using a piece of a lioness's womb as an amulet; and having the woman hold her breath during male orgasm.

Two recipes that appear in classical times persisted throughout the following centuries—making a tea from the bark or leaves of non-fruit-bearing plants (like the willow), and drinking water in which a smith has cooled his tongs. Tea from willow bark was believed to keep a woman from bearing fruit, while smithy's water was meant to sterilize a woman.

The Greeks were the first people to mention a woman's "safe period," when she would not conceive. They believed that when a woman felt sexual desire, she would conceive. Since women were thought to be most aroused just before and after menstruation, the Greeks called those days "unsafe." Although we now know there is no entirely safe period, these are the days with the *least* chance of conception.

The Romans were the first to speak of vinegar as a substance that could prevent conception; its acidity can kill sperm. A man was meant to put it on his penis before intercourse, though this particular use is quite ineffective. Especially interesting is the possibility that the Romans knew of a primitive condom (a sheath that fits over a man's penis and contains the semen). This early condom, made from a goat's bladder, is mentioned in a classical account of the myth of King Minos and his wife, Pasiphaë. If it was available to the Romans, scholars believe it was used only by wealthy aristocrats.

In spite of the physicians' writings, contraception was not widely known or practiced by the Greeks and Romans. The texts were hard to come by, and most women could not read. For most people, abortion and infanticide were the only ways to control family size. The Greeks practiced infanticide at times, leaving babies on temple steps or in wild places. Baby girls were killed more often than boys, as would be expected in a warrior society that valued men more highly than women. Abortion was performed in Greece, probably by using a sharp instrument. Aristotle favored early abortion and drew a line between when a fetus feels life and when it doesn't. He believed that ending a pregnancy was not acceptable after the fetus was alive. Most of the classical writers preferred contraception to abortion, as it was safer for the woman.

Much of the Greeks' medical information reached Arabian and Persian physicians and scholars of the 10th century. Islamic law did not forbid contraception and, in fact, encouraged it by writing about it. Islamic physicians also recognized that certain women should not bear children. In this category they included women with "uterine erosions" (cancer?); women with small uteri; sick women; those with a history of difficult childbearing; and girls who were too young.

Magical remedies had their place, of course. Among them were eating beans on an empty stomach; jumping backward seven times (seven was considered a magic number); taking a child's tooth, wrapping it in a silver leaf, and carrying it. And an old recipe, elephant dung, made a reappearance—it, too, was used by the Egyptians.

Side by side with the magical prescriptions were some more useful ways to block conception: withdrawal (recommended in the writings of the Prophet); preventing male ejaculation (presumably by pressure on the urethra); blocking the cervix with different substances; and putting primitive spermicides on the penis.

Abortion was not forbidden by Islamic law, for the fetus was not held to be a person until it looked like a human being. Effective ways of inducing abortion were known and discussed, along with the belief that "Joking too is useful"![3] (Violent laughter was meant to expel the fetus.)

The concern with women's health, the recognition that childbearing can be harmful, and the open discussion of contraception are distinguishing marks of Islam.

In Europe during the Middle Ages, the climate was entirely different. The great power of the Christian Medieval Church, the emphasis on spirit over body, and the lack

---

[3] Ibid., p. 138.

of support for scientific and medical knowledge that conflicted with Church teachings led to a profound ignorance about contraception. What was known and passed on from person to person included magical charms, herbal teas, and amulets.

One philosopher/alchemist believed that spitting thrice in a frog's mouth and eating bees would keep a woman from becoming pregnant. "Take ye a foot from a live female weasel and tie it round your waist," were the reassuring words of the same philosopher. When philosophers and scholars with access to books and writing were so ignorant of conception and how to prevent it, how could ordinary medieval people know better?

Women had to rely on herbal teas of parsley or lavender; closing doors and locks to close their wombs; drinking water where a smith cooled his tongs; and wearing a salamander's heart round the knee to prevent conception. A medieval woman might be advised to go to her sister's grave and cry out three times (three is a magic number). "No more children, no more!" Or if a bride desired to be four years without children, she could sit down on her hand with four fingers spread out.

These folk beliefs persisted for many centuries, some well into the 1800's. It is incredible that such remedies could last so long in face of the evidence. For child after child must have been born in spite of the teas, charms, weasels' feet, and smithy's water.

By the 17th and 18th centuries in Europe, a new device had appeared, something that would revolutionize the history of contraception—the condom. If the Romans were aware of the condom, that knowledge was lost until the 1500's when one physician, Fallopius, devised a linen sheath to protect men from venereal disease. (Syphilis was epidemic throughout Europe from the late 15th to the early 16th centuries.) His invention was not widespread, and it wasn't until the 17th and 18th centuries that more people knew about and used the condom. Again, it was better known for its protection against venereal disease than for its ability to prevent pregnancy. However, Casanova, the famous libertine of the 1700's, speaks of wearing the condom to block conception. In that age, condoms were made of animal membranes, and the madames of the time did a brisk business selling them to their customers.

When people discovered how to make rubber in 1844, the new condom was more effective, cheaper, and much more widely used. For the first time, ordinary people had access to effective contraception, not just teas, charms, and quackery. Some social crusaders of the early and mid-1800's distributed handbills telling people of ways to prevent conception. They mentioned withdrawal, the use of a sponge soaked in lemon juice, douching with a vinegar solution, and the condom. Contraception became a social and an economic issue as reformers urged people to limit their families and break out of poverty.

In the late 1800's, the rubber cervical cap (a small, cup-shaped device that fits closely over the cervix and prevents sperm from entering) was invented, as was the diaphragm. Now women could control their fertility in a reliable, safe way. Yet contraceptives were still hard to get, and doctors were reluctant to advise their patients on practical methods. It was men and women working outside the medical establishment who made contraceptive information and methods available to people. Annie Besant, working in England in the late 1800's, published a pamphlet which was widely distributed and had great influence. In it, she recommended specific techniques to "check" pregnancy, including the cervical cap. In America, Margaret Sanger opened her first birth control clinic in Brownsville, New York, in 1916. There she advised women on how to prevent pregnancy. Because of the laws forbidding people to give out contraceptive information, her clinic was closed. It was not until many years later that those laws were repealed—largely through Margaret Sanger's work. In 1921, in England, Marie Stopes founded the Society for Constructive Birth Control, which gave out reliable information. When different firms discovered the profit involved in marketing birth control, many devices were advertised in magazines and papers, and sold from door to door. The crusading efforts of reformers were vital in changing attitudes toward birth control, but commercial distribution was equally important. By the end of the first World War, contraceptives were widely accepted and used.

In the years after World War I up to the present, many new contraceptives were developed—some completely unimaginable two generations ago. The plastic I.U.D. (intrauterine device) was improved and became generally known in the 1960's. An egg can still be fertilized in a woman wearing an I.U.D., but the plastic loop or coil does keep the fertilized ovum from attaching itself to the uterine lining, and so prevents pregnancy. It is about 98 percent effective. The Pill, which became well known in the 1960's, is the most famous of recent contraceptive discoveries. Synthetic hormones suppress ovulation in a woman taking the Pill, and the method is almost 100 percent effective. However, because of some potentially dangerous side effects, both the Pill and the I.U.D. are being questioned by women and doctors. The Pill increases the risk of blood clots, while the coil or loop seems related to uterine infections. Both methods must *only* be used under the advice and direction of a doctor.

Sterilization is another form of contraception that is being more widely used today, usually by couples who are through with childbearing. It is a decision not to be made lightly, as sterilization is almost always irreversible. A woman may have her Fallopian tubes severed so no sperm can reach the fertile ovum, or a man can have his sperm ducts sealed off (a vasectomy). Both methods are basically safe and almost 100 percent effective.

We think ourselves a modern, advanced culture, but curiously enough, many of the contraceptive methods in use today have a long and continued history. The condom, vaginal suppositories, chemical spermicides, douches, a small sponge soaked in spermicide, and withdrawal all come from our past. Their present effectiveness is better than olive oil, honey, or alum, but the techniques are much the same. The unsafe period (that the Greeks guessed about) has been correctly identified for *some* women. It is put at the tenth through seventeenth days after the start of a menstrual period, *if* a woman's cycle is a regular twenty-eight days.[4] Since most women's cycles are often irregular, this is not a very reliable method. However, new developments may make the rhythm method more effective. Recent discoveries will help women to pinpoint their time of ovulation—the time to avoid intercourse.

Future advances in contraception include some interesting possibilities. Swedish and American scientists are trying to develop a pill that will prevent semen from penetrating the ovum. Another method involves developing antibodies to sperm, so that a woman would actually be immunized against pregnancy. However, the emphasis is still on women taking major responsibility for birth control. Scientists continue to focus on synthetic hormones that will interrupt a woman's ovulatory cycle—a questionable method. More research needs to be done on safe and reliable contraception for *both* men and women.

It has been a long and fumbling development from elephant dung to the I.U.D. Often people have been pathetically wrong about how to prevent conception. But if we've left behind the herbal teas, weasels' feet, and salamanders' hearts, we've also kept many of the basic contraceptive techniques. One theme unites the long search for effective contraception—men's and women's age-old desire to control their fertility, to have children only when they choose.

---

[4] Roberts Rugh and Landrum B. Shettles, *From Conception to Birth* (New York: Harper & Row, 1971), p. 186.

Chapter 12
"HOW TO GET A CHILD"

The souls of babies rest in the wild fig trees where green pigeons roost, according to one culture. Another thought spirit children hid behind special stones waiting for young, desirable women to pass by. Yet another believed that tiny children lived curled up within the male sperm.

What people believe about conception influences what they do to "get" a child. If souls rest in trees, women might "call" them from the leaves. If spirit babies hide behind sacred rocks, women must visit such places. In recorded history there are as many ways to get with child as there are medicines in a drugstore. But in the past, the living world was people's pharmacy and magic their medicine. When a woman desired a child, there were many remedies she could try.[1] Most of the cures for barrenness or ways to become pregnant are based on this belief: the world is full of fertility, a quantity that can be gathered and used.

Certain trees and plants were thought to help women to bear because they produce fruit, nuts, and berries (the "children" of the plant). In Northern India, barren women went to a sacred palm and picked a coconut to help them become pregnant. Another group of Indian women visited an apple tree and rolled on the ground beneath it to soak up the bearing power of the tree. A woman from Yugoslavia who wanted children would take a chemise and put it on a fruit-bearing tree on the night before St. George's day. Overnight, it was believed to absorb the

---

[1] In general, it was assumed to be the woman's fault if she did not conceive, and cures for barrenness were directed toward her.

special productivity of the tree. The next morning the woman took down her chemise and put it on, placing that magical "fruitfulness" close to her body.

In ancient Rome, women gathered under the wild fig in midsummer to honor Juno, the goddess of women. They took up sticks and hit each other in a mock fight, "beating" the fertility of the fig tree into each other.

Other plants that produce berries and grain were believed to give their fruitfulness to women. A tea made from mistletoe, which has clusters of poisonous, pale berries, was thought to cure sterility among medieval women. At a medieval wedding, girls who walked before the bride carried wreaths of wheat to make the marriage productive. A Greek bride held a pomegranate in her hand when she went to her new home, hoping the fruit's many seeds would give her many children. The wedding party that followed showered her with nuts for the same purpose, just as some Indian peoples threw rice at their brides.

Any creature that bore many young would help women to have children, some people believed. In the last century, women of an Indian tribe on Vancouver Island drank a special tea made from flies' feet or wasps' nests so they might breed as successfully as did those insects. Using the same idea, a White Mountain Apache woman might eat the eggs of a certain spider to relieve her barrenness.

Animals could also give women the ability to bear young, according to certain cultures. Goats were often used in fertility rites, as the male was known for his sexual ardor. In the ancient rite of the Lupercalia, the boundaries of Rome were magically redrawn each spring. Two young men, called he-goats, were smeared with blood from sacrificed goats. Stripped almost naked and holding pieces of the animals' hides, they ran the boundaries of Rome. A man or woman desiring children stood by the city's edge, for the he-goats struck anyone they saw with a strip of goat hide. This rite "beat" fertility into a man or woman and also made a magic circle around the powers of good luck and fruitfulness, shutting out evil and sterility.

Because gophers breed prolifically, a Walapai Indian woman might cut off the animal's foot, boil and eat it. Then she would have as many sons and daughters as the gopher.

Snakes were also linked with human fertility, as they were a symbol for the penis. This symbolism is so ancient that figurines dating to 6,000 B.C., have been found of a pregnant goddess with a carved snake winding around her abdomen. Surely, this was a potent charm for the fertility of men and women, as well as fields and crops.

Another kind of magic believed to produce children involved dolls or images representing an infant. Among one Indian tribe of California, friends of a barren woman made a doll from grass and put it in a carrying basket. This they put in the woman's hut. When she entered, the woman took up the "baby," put it to her breast, and sang lullabies. The magic of having a pretend child was meant to give her a real one. Using a similar charm, a woman of West Africa carried a wooden doll on her back, just as women did their live infants. But in Japan, the rites were more elaborate. There, the old women of the village visited the house of a woman who wanted children. As serious as any real midwives, they mimed the delivery of a baby, holding up a doll at the end.

Among many peoples the mandrake root was thought to relieve sterility because the roots somewhat resemble a human being. In Genesis, Reuben gathered mandrakes to help his mother bear more children. Hundreds of years later, medieval Europeans still thought the root would help women conceive. The idea behind all these charms and rites is this: if a woman carries, nurses, or delivers something resembling a child, that will magically bring her a live baby.

For other peoples, "getting" a child is bound up with the myths of the country and with complex beliefs about the origin of souls. Some cultures believe the souls of babies rest in sacred places—stones, trees, or hills. The Aborigine tribes of the Great Victoria Desert in Australia thought there were places created long ago by the mythical ancestors where spirit babies gathered. A person might see them from a distance as they warmed themselves by the fire. A woman could go to a spirit center and sit down with her legs open, hoping a child would enter her body or follow her home. In North Arnhem Land, Australia, the Aborigines believed children were linked to sacred wells and took the form of fish or animals. A man might catch such a soul and bring it back to his wife, "putting" it in her body.

The American Hidatsa Indians thought the souls of infants lived in certain "baby hills." Inside they looked like hogans (earth-covered lodges), where old men cared for the children. To get with child, a wife left toys at the foot of the hill, trying to persuade a spirit baby to come home with her. Or a man could fast there to gain sons.

Some Eskimos told of the souls of children who waited on top of the cold snow. If a woman passed by with her boot strings undone, a spirit could climb up her laces into her body.

Live children themselves might be used to bring fertility to women. At the weddings of some European Slavs and some women of India, people put a small boy in the bride's lap so she, too, would have sons. A Baiga woman of India followed a different custom, taking the umbilical cord from a newborn and tying it in a cloth. She wore the powerful charm next to her body, believing it would bring a baby to her.

It is not just the living who are thought to give fertility; some people think the dead can cure sterility and make women pregnant. Because the dead "live" in the fruitful earth that yields crops and food, they are believed to partake of this bearing power. For the Nyakyusa of Africa, "the shade and the semen are brothers." [2] The dead ancestors control conception in their living relatives. If a woman does not conceive, it may be because the shades are

---

[2] Monica Wilson, "Nyakyusa Ritual and Symbolism," in *Myth and Cosmos,* ed. by John Middleton (Garden City, N.J.: The Natural History Press, 1967), p. 158.

angry with her. To appease the dead, a bull is sacrificed when a girl reaches puberty; then the shades will not make her sterile when she marries.

In Yugoslavia years ago, a woman would visit the grave of a dead pregnant woman. Calling out her name, the barren wife prayed for children. Then she took a bit of earth from the grave and wore it next to her body, hoping to absorb the power of the bearing one.

Other people believe the dead are born again in new children. The Tlinglit Indians took a fingernail or lock of hair from a loved dead person and gave it to a girl of the same clan. She carried the nail or bit of hair in her belt, believing her relative would be reborn in her child.

Yet fertility is not a quantity that flows endlessly through the world. For many, it is seen as limited, while others feel it can be threatened or made powerless. The African Nyakyusa believe that the fertility in the world is of a fixed amount. When a girl reaches puberty, her parents must not have any new children until she is safely married. (This happens soon after puberty.) One part of the tribe even forbids parents to make love until the marriage is completed. Their fertility would take away from hers, making the girl sterile.

The Romans believed in a kind of power they called *numen*, which gods, beasts, human beings, and the earth shared. A woman who bore children had it, as did a cow who bore a calf. It was a power that could give out, be used up, and it must be magically replenished by the proper sacrifices and offerings, lest women stop bearing and cows stop producing their young.

In medieval times, it was a common belief that fertility diminished a man's life-span. There was only so much power within a man, and when he gave life to a child through conception, he lost years of his own. So the poet, John Donne, wrote, "We kill ourselves to propagate our kind." [3]

---

[3] Leonard Dean, ed., *Renaissance Poetry,* 2nd edition (Englewood Cliffs, N.J.: Prentice-Hall, 1964), p. 225.

Other people feel that evil and fertility are in conflict, that good spirits give many children and abundant crops, while bad spirits give sterility and death. One way for women to be fruitful, then, is to drive away the evil spirits who delight in spreading barrenness and blighting the land. In one tribe of West Africa, the men protected women from the demon of sterility by firing guns and waving sharp swords.

Evil ones also seem to hate jokes and laughter, especially sexual jokes and gestures. It was the custom at Greek and Roman weddings for the party to make broad jokes about the married pair. This would drive off the powers of bad luck and infertility. The Elizabethans also told ribald jokes after a wedding, while today, a newly married couple may still be teased about their wedding night.

On the evening before the marriage of a Gurkha man and woman (of the Himalayas), the women gathered at the bride-to-be's house. There they danced and sang, told wild jokes, and mimed the act of making love. All this was to bring good luck and children to the married pair.

Intercourse, itself, could be seen as a powerful rite that drove off sterility and brought fertility to men and women, their fields, and their animals. In ancient Greece, a couple ritually made love in a freshly plowed field at the time of the autumn sowing. It was a magical act to bring fruitfulness to all living things.

Probably the most common and widespread way to "get" a child was to ask for one, praying to the right goddess and making offerings. Remember the abundant goddess of the last Ice Age? A barren woman might have prayed to her for children or worn a necklace of small ivory breasts to make her pregnant. Egyptian women had several birth goddesses they could pray to, including Taueret, who was portrayed as a hippopotamus with breasts. The Greeks made offerings to Artemis (goddess of the moon and of children) and Eileithyia, often shown kneeling as if giving birth. Roman women prayed to Juno, goddess of women, who was also linked to the moon. Because many people connected the waxing of the moon with the swelling of a pregnant woman, birth goddesses were often moon goddesses. As such, they were concerned with women, for the cycles of a woman's body closely follow the cycles of the moon.

Many cultures throughout history have prayed to goddesses who were primarily seen as mothers. Chinese women left offerings at the temple of the "Mother," while women of India asked for children from Shashthi, the "sixth mother." In our own culture, the figure most closely connected with the old Mother Goddess is the Virgin Mary. While not worshipped as a goddess, "The Mother of God" is seen by some Christians as a powerful being—one who can answer prayers for children and who is directly involved with women's lives. Remember Queen Anne who visited every Notre Dame (dedicated to the Virgin Mary) in France as she prayed for an heir?

Most cultures had a goddess who gave women children and then protected them in birth. Often she was linked to the moon and to the sowing of the fields. It is an ancient comparison—the sown field with the pregnant woman—and ceremonies meant to give fertility to the fields were also believed to make children grow within women.

It seems we have moved a long way from the old rites, the ancient charms. When we think of a woman today who desires children and can't have them, we think of doctors, sterility clinics, medical treatment. But are we so far away from the Indians and their rice, or the Roman wedding party with its ribald jokes?

At a modern wedding, people throw rice at the bride—a custom whose meaning we've lost. We're really "throwing" fertility at the woman when we shower her with rice. In her hand the bride often carries a bouquet of flowers surrounded by Baby's Breath, while little children may be part of the wedding procession. The Baby's Breath and children can be seen as good luck charms for the woman's future fertility. The traditional bride still wears something blue, a color used in past times to repel the evil eye—the evil associated with bad luck and sterility. The wedding ring itself, while it has other meanings, is like the sacred circle that shuts in fertility and good luck. People still make jokes after a wedding, and some are fairly broad. The Romans laughed bad luck and infertility away from their brides; we do the same. When it comes time for the married pair to leave, they drive off with tin cans rattling behind. Evil powers hate loud noises; and though we may not realize it, we are scaring ill luck away.

The old comparison between a fertile field and a woman is also part of our culture. When we speak of conception we talk of a man's "seed" and "the fruit of the womb," while a miscarriage may be the result of a "bad seed."

We are part of the past, just as the past is part of us. The echoes of Greek and Roman celebrations are with us when we rejoice at a wedding; the bride with a pomegranate in her hand is still near to us; and the gay celebrants with their noisy jokes are heard in our rites. Our clothes do not resemble ancient ones, our charms don't sound like charms, and the words we use to ask for children are different. But we still call on the powers of fertility, we wear magic circles to shut out bad luck, and many brides continue to marry in June, the month sacred to Juno, goddess of women and childbirth.

Glossary

GLOSSARY

Accoucheur—The French word for the doctor who attends at birth; literally, "he who is present at the bedside." [1]

Afterbirth—The strong, flexible membranes that surround the child within the uterus, through which the child receives nourishment, and which is delivered through the vagina soon after the baby is born. The afterbirth is connected to the child's navel by the umbilical cord.

After pains—Contractions that continue after the birth is over, and which help reduce the size of the uterus.

Amniotic fluid—A watery liquid that cushions the baby inside the placenta. Some time before delivery, the sac containing the fluid breaks and the liquid flows through the vagina.

Amniotic sac—The inner membrane of the placenta, which encloses the amniotic fluid and the baby.

Bag of waters—Another term for the amniotic sac. People speak of the bag of waters "breaking" when the amniotic sac ruptures and releases its fluid.

Birth—The actual expulsion of a baby from the uterus, through the vagina, and out of the woman's body.

Birth canal—A term for the combined length of the open uterus and the vagina during the actual passage of the baby.

Birth fluids—Same as amniotic fluid.

Birth stool—A low seat on which a woman sits, stands, or crouches to deliver the baby. Usually, a U-shaped area is cut out of the stool's seat to allow passage of the baby.

Breech birth—Delivery of the child bottom-first. It is often more difficult for the mother than a normal, head-first birth.

---

[1] Jess Stein and Laurence Urdang, eds., *The Random House Dictionary* (New York: Random House, 1966), p. 9.

Caul—A section of the amniotic sac that occasionally covers a baby's head at birth. In past times, a caul was thought to be a sign of good luck and a protection against drowning.

Cervix—The tapering end of a woman's uterus that projects into the vagina. It widens and stretches during labor to approximately 10 cm, to allow the baby's head and body to pass through.

Conception—When an egg is fertilized by a sperm and the resulting mass of cells successfully implants in the uterus; the act of becoming pregnant.

Contraception—The act of preventing conception by mechanical or chemical means.

Contraction—An involuntary pulling of the uterine muscles which acts to widen the cervix and finally expel the baby. In early labor, contractions are usually painless, while in the later stages of labor, they can be painful; traditionally called "pains."

Crowning—When the top of the baby's head appears at and stretches the opening of the vagina.

Demerol—A mild narcotic used to kill pain and frequently given to women during the first stage of labor.

Due date—The time (calculated by a pregnant woman and her doctor) predicting when the baby will be born. It is decided by adding ten days to the first day of the last menstrual period, subtracting three months, and adding one year.

Embryo—The earliest stage of the developing baby inside the uterus, up to the third month of life.

Ejaculation—Male orgasm, when sperm are released from the penis.

Episiotomy—The small cut made in the flesh behind the vulva, meant to reduce ragged tearing in women as they give birth. American doctors routinely perform episiotomies, while many European doctors do not.

Fallopian tubes—The two narrow tubes (4″ long) leading from a woman's ovaries to her uterus. The egg passes from the ovary to a Fallopian tube, where it may be fertilized, and then travels to the uterus.

Fertile period—That time in a woman's menstrual cycle when the egg can be fertilized (usually lasting about two-three days). For additional safety, in women using the rhythm method, it is put between the tenth and seventeenth days after the start of a menstrual period in a woman with a regular 28-day cycle.

Fetus—The developing baby within the uterus from the third month to birth.

Fraternal twins—Two babies that grow from two separate eggs fertilized by two different sperms. Usually, fraternal twins have two separate placentas.

Identical twins—Two babies that usually develop from one egg fertilized by one sperm. The fertilized ovum then splits in two. The babies share the same placenta but normally have different amniotic sacs inside.

Labor—The process from the first regular contractions to birth.

First stage labor—When contractions gradually stretch the cervix from a tiny opening to one about ten cm in diameter. It can last seven–thirteen hours or more, depending on whether it's a first birth.

Second stage labor—The amniotic sac often breaks now, and the baby passes through the cervix, down the vaginal canal, and is born. In a normal birth, it lasts from one-half hour to about two hours.

Third stage labor—The placenta is delivered, sometimes a few minutes after birth up to one-half hour later.

Lamaze method—A technique for controlling the pain of childbirth through different types of breathing. (Named after the French doctor, Fernand Lamaze.)

Leboyer, Frederick—The French doctor who feels present delivery methods are harsh and traumatic to newborns. He advocates a dim, quiet delivery room, putting the baby on the mother's stomach immediately after birth, and then washing the child in warm water.

Lightening—When the baby's head drops lower in the pelvic area in preparation for birth. It usually happens a few weeks before birth.

Lochial fluids—A combination of blood and other liquids that flow gradually from a woman's uterus after birth. The discharge may last from one to three weeks.

Lying-in couch—A special low, narrow bed designed for childbearing.

Menstrual cycle—A time period covering these things: the gradual preparation of a soft lining within the uterus; the release of a mature egg from the ovaries; an egg's journey through the Fallopian tubes to the uterus; and the shedding of the lining and egg, if unfertilized, as menstrual fluid at the end.

Midwife—From the early English *midwif,* meaning "with

woman." A woman who attends the mother during birth.

Multiple births—The delivery of more than one child after labor.

Obstetrician—A doctor trained in prenatal care, childbirth, and care after delivery.

Ovaries—Two small (walnut-sized) organs located near a woman's uterus that contain undeveloped eggs and produce a mature one monthly. They also secrete the female sex hormones, estrogen and progesterone.

Ovum—The mature egg, or female reproductive cell, as it is released from the ovaries and enters the Fallopian tubes.

Penis—The male sexual organ.

Placenta—The thick sac of tissues and blood vessels across which nutrients pass to the baby and waste products pass to the mother's blood-stream. It contains the amniotic sac and baby and is the same as afterbirth.

Post-partum depression—A mood change sometimes experienced by women a few days after birth and usually lasting several days to a few weeks. It is thought to be caused by hormonal changes in the body after delivery.

Puerperium—The time after delivery up to eight weeks, when a woman's uterus is returning to normal size (about that of a fist).

Quickening—When the movements of the fetus within the womb are first felt by the mother; usually occurs in the fifth month of pregnancy. In past times, people thought this was when the fetus came to life.

Rooming-in—The hospital practice of allowing newborns to stay and sleep in their mother's room. It seems to help in forming the mother-child bond and is especially convenient for mothers who breast-feed their infants.

Safe period—That time during a woman's monthly cycle when she is unable to conceive, either because the egg has not yet been released or because it is too "old" to be fertilized. Usually put from the first day of menstruation through the ninth day, and then the eighteenth through twenty-eighth day, in a regular 28-day cycle.

Sperm—The male reproductive cell, shaped like a tiny bead with a fine tail. Sperm are continuously produced inside a man's testicles and are released through the penis during ejaculation.

Sperm ducts—(Technically, vas deferens.) The two tubes which carry sperm from a man's testicles to the base of his penis.

Trimester—A three-month span of time. Pregnancy is divided into three trimester periods.

Twilight sleep—A term describing the heavily anesthetized state of women during childbirth; favored by obstetricians during the 1940's.

Umbilical cord—The tube that stretches from the baby's navel to the placenta. Through it pass blood vessels carrying nutrients and oxygen to the fetus.

Urethra—The narrow tube that extends to the tip of the penis, through which urine and semen can (separately) pass.

Uterus—The muscular bag about the size of a fist inside a woman's pelvic cavity. Inside, the fertilized ovum implants in the lining and grows into a fetus.

Vagina—The inner sexual organ of a woman; the muscular canal (about 3¾" long) leading from the vulva to just beyond the cervix.

Vasectomy—A small operation in which a man's sperm ducts are cut and tied so no sperm can reach the penis.

Vernix—The white waxy substance (composed of dead skin cells) that may cover a baby's skin at birth. It seems to help the infant resist skin infections if it is rubbed in and not washed off.

Vulva—The outer sexual organs of a woman, through which the baby is delivered.

Wet nurse—A woman who is employed to breast-feed another's baby. She, herself, must have had a child recently.

Womb—Same as uterus.

For Further Reading

FOR FURTHER READING *

Berndt, R. M. and C. H. Berndt, *The World of the First Australians.* Chicago: University of Chicago Press, 1965.
Calas, Nicolas and Margaret Mead, eds., *Primitive Heritage.* New York: Random House, 1953.
Coon, Carleton S., *The Hunting Peoples.* Boston: Little, Brown and Company, 1971, also paperback, 1972.
Crump, Lucy, *Nursery Life 300 Years Ago.* New York: E. P. Dutton and Company, 1930.
Cushing, Frank, *My Adventures in Zuñi.* Sante Fe: The Peripatetic Press, 1941.
Doolittle, Rev. Justus, *Social Life of the Chinese,* vol. 1. New York: Harper & Brothers, Publishers, 1867.
Drucker, Philip, *Indians of the Northwest Coast, the Northern and Central Nootkan Tribes,* Smithsonian Institute, Bureau of American Ethnology, Bull. no. 144. Washington D. C.: U. S. Government Printing Office, 1951.
Frazer, Sir James George, *The New Golden Bough,* abridged and edited by Dr. Theodor H. Gaster. New York: Criterion Books, 1959, and New American Library, paperback, 1975.
Freuchen, Peter, *Adventures in the Arctic,* ed. by Dagmar Freuchen. Cleveland: World Publishing Company, 1960.
Freuchen, Peter, *Book of the Eskimos,* ed. by Dagmar Freuchen. Cleveland: World Publishing Company, 1961.
Headland, Issac T., *Home LIfe in China.* New York: The Macmillan Company, 1914.
Himes, Norman E., *Medical History of Contraception.* New York: Schocken Books, paperback, 1970.
Marshack, Alexander, *The Roots of Civilization.* New York: McGraw-Hill Book Company, 1972.

* These books are necessarily adult titles, as that is what's available.

Mead, Margaret, *Male and Female*. New York: Dell Publishing Co., paperback, 1968.

Mead, Margaret, *Sex and Temperament in Three Primitive Societies*. New York: William Morrow and Co., 1935.

Middleton, John, ed., *Myth and Cosmos*. Garden City: The Natural History Press, 1967.

Pomeroy, Sarah B., *Goddessess, Whores, Wives, Slaves*. New York: Schocken Books, 1975.

Rose, H.J., *Religion in Greece and Rome*. New York: Harper and Row, 1959, also paperback.

Scheinfeld, Amram, *Twins and Supertwins*. New York: J. P. Lippincott Company, 1967.

Stevenson, Matilda C., "The Zuñi Indians," 23rd Annual Report of the Bureau of American Ethnology. Washington D.C. : U. S. Government Printing Office, 1904.

Wolf, John B., *Louis XIV*. New York: W. W. Norton and Company, 1968.

Index

INDEX

Abandonment, 12, 17, 26, 35, 36-37
Aborigine, 86, 108, 110, 121-22
Abortion, 110, 111, 113, 114
Accoucheur, see Doctors, of childbirth
Africa:
  Nyakyusa tribe, 81-86, 122, 123
  other tribes, 87, 88, 109, 121, 124
  Yoruba, 86-87
Afterbirth, 7, 15, 26-27, 36, 49, 59, 68, 77, 82, 102, 122
America, 87, 88, 93-103, 116, 118
Amniotic sac, 47, ff. 47, 95
Amulets, 4, 5, 37, 107, 108, 112, 113, 114, 115
Ancestors, 8, 57, 61, 81, 82
Arapesh, see New Guinea
Archaeology, 3-8
Aristotle, 112, 113-114
Art and artifacts, 3-5, 7, 87

Baby, see Newborn
Bag of water, see Amniotic sac
Baptism, 69
Barrenness, 11-13, 55, 56, 64, 65, 108, 109, 113, ff. 119, 120, 122, 123, 124, 125
Bathing, ritual:
  of child, 50-51, 52, 60, 68, 84, 97
  of father, 29
  of mother, 51, 52, 84, 102
  of shaman, 79

Besant, Annie, 116
Betrothal, 23-24, 60
Bible, 88, 112, 121
Birth:
  abnormal, 95, 96
  attendants, 7, 76, 82
  beds, 66, 82, 101
  blood, 5, 6, 15, 17, 25, 28, 29, 82
  clinics, 116
  control, see Contraception
  hut, 5, 7, 25-26, 27, 76
  opening, see Vulva
  position, 5, 6-7, 14, 26, 35, 48, 58, 67-68, 76, 82, 101
  stool, 14, 98
  witnesses, 67, 69
Blood-letting, 31, 65-66
Breast-feeding, see Nursing
Breathing, controlled, see Lamaze
Breech birth, 87

Carvings, see Art and artifacts
Casanova, 115-116
Ceremony, see Rites
Cervix, 109, 111, 112, 114
"Children of God," 88, 89
China, 55-61, 97, 98, 125
Circle, magic, 120, 125-126
Conception, 6, 24, 64-65, 81, 107, 108, 110, 111, 115, 119, 122, 123, 126
Contraception:
  abstinence, 110
  cervical cap, 116

141

condom, 113, 115-116, 117
diaphragm, 116
douche, 110, 112, 117
Intrauterine Device, 117
Pill, the, 117
rhythm method, 118
safe period, 113, 117
spermicide, 110, 111, 112, 113, 114, 117
withdrawal, 111, 112, 114, 117
Contraction, 99, 100
Cro-Magnon, 3, 108

Daughters:
American, 102
Arapesh, 31
Chinese, 59-61
Eskimo, 35
Greek, ff. 18, 26, 113
Nootka, 77
Nyakusa, 82
Zuñi, 44, 48-52
Dauphin, 64, 65, 66, 68-71
Dead, the, 8, 11, 81, 82, 83, 85, 109, 122, 123
Dean, Leonard, ff. 123
Delivery, 7, 13, 14-15, 26, 35, 48, 58, 68, 76-77, 82, 101-102
room, 101
Divorce, 56, 64
Doctors, 112, 113, 114, 115, 116, 117, 125
of childbirth, 65, 66, 94, 95, 96, 98, 100-102
Donne, John, 123
Drugs, *see* Medication

Egyptians, 111-112, 124
Embryo, 95
England, 97, 116
Episiotomy, 101, 102
Eskimo, 6, 33-39, 86, 98, 122
Europe, 97, 114, 115, 121, 122
Evil:
eye, 15, 18, 125

spirits, 16, 56, 57, 60, 120, 124, 126

Fallopius, 115
Family, 7, 11-12, 17, 18, 28, 29-31, 34-38, 45-52, 56, 60, 61, 76-78, 82, 94
Father (husband), 4, 6, 7, 11, 12, 13, 15, 16, 17-18, 23, 24-32, 35-36, 44, 45, 52, 55, 60, 68, 75, 83, 94, 96-97, 98, 99
"Fearful Ones", *see* Twin parents
Fertility, 4, 12, 13, 37, 49, 50, 55-56, 64, 87, 108, 116, 118, 119-126
Fetus, 95, 114
Fifth-day ceremony, 16, 17, 19
Fire, sacred, *see* Hearth
Foot-binding, 61
France, 3, 63-71
Future, foretelling of, 11, 56, 60, 69, 87

Gift-giving, ritual, 18, 30, 47, 60
Goddesses, birth:
Chinese, 55, 57, 61, 107, 125
Christian, 4, 64, 66, 125
Greek, 11, 12, 13, 14, 15, 124
Ice Age, 3-6, 7, 8, 124
Prehistory, 121
Roman, 120, 124, 126
Twin, 86
Zuñi, 44
Gods, 17-18, 32, 50, 51, 69
Greece, 11-19, 89, 98, 112-114, 117, 120, 124, 126

Halliday, William R., ff. 17
Hearth, sacred, 5, 6, 17
Hebrews, ancient, 112
Herbs:
for birth, 14, 46, 49, 51, 67
for conception, 119, 120, 121, 125, 126

142

for contraception, 108-114
for protection, 27
for purification, 29
Home birth, 97
Hospital, 96-103
Husband, see Father
Hypnosis, 96

Ice Age, 3-8, 124
India, 119, 120, 122, 125
Indians:
    American, 109, 120, 121, 122, 123
    Nootka, 7, 75-79, 86, 87-88
    Zuñi, 43-52
Infanticide, 86, 110, 113
Infant mortality, 98, 108
Intercourse, ritual, 85, 124
Islam, 114
Isolation huts, 27, 78, 83-85

Japan, 88, 121

Labor, 6-7, 14, 25-26, 28, 34-35, 45-48, 57-58, 66-68, 82, 99-101
Labor pain, see Contraction
Labor room, 99
Lamaze method, 96, 98, 99, 102
Leboyer method, 96
Legitimacy, 18, 19
Louis XIII, 63, 64, 68
Louis XIV, 69, 71
Lunar cycle, 3-4, 124-125
Lying-in couch, see Birth beds

Malaurie, Jean, ff. 39
Marriage, 13, 24, 60, 61, 63, 88, 123, 124, 125
Marshack, Alexander, 3-4, 5
Mead, Margaret, ff. vii, 5, ff. 28, ff. 29
Medication, 95, 96, 98, 100

Medicine woman, 84-85, 109
Medieval, see Middle Ages
Menstrual cycle, 5, 24, 25, 113, 117-118, 125
Middle Ages, 114-115, 120, 121, 123
Midwife, 14, 15, 46-51, 57, 58, 59, 66-68, 97, 109, 110
Minos, king, myth, 113
Morning sickness, 95
Multiple births, 75-89

Naming, 7-8, 17-18, 19, 31, 37, 59, 60, 69
Neanderthal, 108
New Guinea, 23-32, 97, 109, 110
Newborn, 7, 30, 38-39, 48-49, 58-59, 76-77, 82, 96, 101, 102, 103
Nootka, see Indians
Nursing, 15, 26, 36, 38, 51, 70, 103, 110, 112

Obstetrician, see Doctors, of childbirth
Ocher, red, 5, 7
Ovulation, 110, 117, 118

Péronne, Dame, 67-68
Physician, see Doctors
Placenta, see Afterbirth
Plato, 112
Pregnancy, 13, 24, 27, 33, 44-45, 55, 65-68, 75, 93-98, 112, 118
Prehistory, see Ice Age
Priests, 18, 48, 58, 69
Puppets, 58, 97, 98

Queen Anne, 63-69, 125
Quickening, 25, ff. 25, 66

143

Rites:
  of baptism, 50-52, 69
  of growth, 12, 28-29, 30-32, 50, 95, 102, 124, 125
  of initiation, 31-32
  of pregnancy, 4, 44, 56, 75, 95
  of protection, 7, 15, 16, 37, 38, 44, 51-52, 56, 57, 60, 66, 102
  of purification, 17, 29, 50-52, 83-85, 102
  of separation, 27-29, 60
  of welcome, 7, 17, 18
Rome, 112-113, 115, 120, 123, 124, 125, 126
Romulus and Remus, 89

Sacrifices, 11, 12, 18, 55, 57, 85, 107, 120, 123, 124
Salmon Spirits, 77, 79
Sanger, Margaret, 116
Sculpture, see Art and artifacts
Shamans, 37, 75, 78, 79, 86
Sons:
  Arapesh, 26, 31, 32
  Chinese, 55-56, 59
  Eskimo, 35, 38
  French, 63, 64, 65, 68
  Greek, 11, 15-19, 113
  Nootka, 76
Soul, 6, 27, 30, 37, 69, 108, 119, 121, 122
South America, 109-110
Sterile sheets, 98, 101, 102
Sterility, see Barrenness
Sterilization, 111, 112, 117
Stopes, Marie, 116
Swaddling, 15, 68, 70

Taboos:
  birth, 14, 16, 25, 27, 59, 60
  growth, 23-24, 28, 30
  intercourse, 24, 30, 55
  nursing, 77

  pregnancy, 25, 55, 56, 75, 81-82, 94, 95
  twin, 77, 78, 82-85
Talmud, 112
Triplets see Multiple births
Twilight sleep, 93
Twin parents, 75-76, 77-79, 83-86, 87, 89
Twins, see Multiple births

Umbilical, see Afterbirth
Uterus, 95, 97, 98, 101, 110, 111, 112, 114

Vacuum bubble, 97
Vasectomy, 117
Venereal disease, 115
Vulva, 4-5, 6, 102

Wedding, see Marriage
Wet-nurse, 70
Wilson, Monica, ff. 81, ff. 84, ff. 122
Witches, 16, 44-45
Womb, see Uterus
Women, Eskimo, 33-39, 98
Women:
  in Africa, 81-86
  in America, 93-103
  in China, 55-61, 97
  in France, 63-71
  in Greece, 11-19, 98
  in Ice Age, 3-8, 124
  in New Guinea, 23-32, 97
Women, Indian:
  Nootka, 75-79
  Zuñi, 43-52, 97

Yoruba, see Africa
Yugoslavia, 119-120, 123

Zuñi, see Indians

144